# Courage to Care

*A Caregiver's Guide Through*
*Each Stage of Alzheimer's*

**Joanne Parrent**

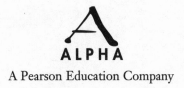

ALPHA

A Pearson Education Company

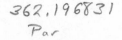
*To my late father, and my mother.*

# Contents at a Glance

## Appendixes

# Contents

# Introduction

When the idea of doing this book was first presented to me by my editor, Mike Sanders, I wondered why there should be another book on Alzheimer's disease. The library and bookstore shelves were filled with books—everything from the popular *36-Hour Day* to books by caregivers about their particular experiences, and even books by patients in the early stage of the disease. What could I contribute to this important subject that wasn't already out there? As I looked deeper, however, I realized that there really wasn't a book that in a clear, simple way took the reader through what he or she would need to know as a caregiver in each stage of the disease. I wanted to create a book that would do just that.

As I began my research, I also thought about what experiences I had to draw on for this book. As a writer, I knew how to research a subject and organize large amounts of material, but I had never had a family member with Alzheimer's disease. I did know others who had been or were currently dealing with the disease in their families. As I spoke to them, I realized that I did have the experience of dealing with dementia in my family and, in some important ways, my experience was similar to those dealing with Alzheimer's.

Several years ago, my father began behaving in a peculiar manner. One day he put the toaster oven in the refrigerator and later had no memory of doing that. He began to get lost in familiar places and had terrible anxiety about being in unfamiliar ones. He refused to travel alone even to visit me and even though my mother would have walked him to the gate of the plane and I would have been there at the other end to meet him. He told me how frustrated he was that he couldn't think of words when he wanted to, how he would forget what he was saying in the middle of a sentence. He confided that he was very worried about what was happening to him. He had been to his doctor and even to the hospital for some tests, but they didn't know what was wrong with him.

Although he never used the frightening words—Alzheimer's disease—I think that was his greatest fear. I wanted him to go to the medical center in nearby Ann Arbor, Michigan, for more tests. Before that could happen, however, he had a massive stroke that left him with symptoms similar to those in the middle stage of Alzheimer's disease. He couldn't speak coherently—he'd talk about things that didn't make sense to us. He made strange, repetitive motions with his hands. He was difficult to manage and even violent at times. Formerly a gentle, easy-going man, he now had frequent outbursts of anger. Six weeks after the stroke, he died.

For those six weeks before he died, my mother, my sister, and I had to cope with—in a short period of time—much of what the families of people diagnosed with AD must cope with over a period of many years. We had to find a doctor who could give us an accurate and truthful diagnosis. We had to accept the fact that his brain damage was irreversible. We had to find a facility to put him in, because my mother couldn't handle him alone and my sister and I lived in other states. We experienced moments when we laughed at the humorous things he said. We felt hope when he had a good day and cried when he had a bad one. We had to think about the financial and legal plans—including how to pay for his long-term care when his Medicare coverage ran out. My mother had to deal with her own increasing caregiver stress as she rushed back and forth to the home every day and tried to make sure that her husband was getting the best possible care. She had to decide whether or not to send him back to the hospital for extraordinary measures after he had a second stroke or to let the staff of the facility give him only comfort care until the end. We all had to go through our own grieving process in our own ways—first grieving the loss of his ability to communicate with us and second his ultimate loss. My mother, in particular, had to build a new life as a single person after almost 50 years of married life.

Writing this book has been a way—after my own family's experience—that I hope I can help others cope with the trauma of dealing with dementia in a loved one. The coping my family had to do in a short six weeks will extend for years or even decades for families dealing with Alzheimer's disease, and that is an even more difficult challenge. We all care when a loved one is stricken with illness, but it takes a special kind of courage to keep on caring year after year—when the person no longer recognizes you and when he is so different from the person he once was. This book cannot give caregivers that courage, but it can arm them with knowledge that will make their journey easier.

Alzheimer's disease is the dying of the light. It's the dying of the electric sparks in the brain that make the connections among nerve cells to enable us to connect to others and to the world at large. For those who develop Alzheimer's disease, the light is slowly going out, the connections are slowing breaking. My hope for now is that this book can light the way for caregivers whose loved ones are gradually descending into that darkness.

And my greatest hope for the future is that, through the courage and compassion of caregivers, combined with the genius of scientists working on the many fronts discussed in the last chapter of this book, one day soon no one will have to lose their connection to a loved because of dementia. One day, we may all be able to say good-bye to those we love, not years before but instead at the very end of life.

# Acknowledgments

Many people have been important in the making of this book. Specifically, I'd like to thank the technical editor, Barbara Bernstein. She not only read the manuscript to make sure the content was accurate, she also shared many stories and provided me with helpful materials during the process of writing the book. Mike Sanders, the acquisitions editor, first conceived of the book. Both he and Debbie Romaine, the development editor, helped shape the final book. Debbie provided thoughtful comments on the manuscript, forcing me to make it better. And no author can be happy without a good, detail-oriented production editor, and Christy Wagner filled that role. I'd like to give an extra-special thanks to my agent and partner, Brenda Feigen. She went beyond the call of duty on this project. She also was very supportive during my long hours of work on the book.

More generally, I'd like to thank all of my friends and new acquaintances who told me stories of their mothers, fathers, or spouses with Alzheimer's disease and their own experiences as caregivers. Finally, I'd like to thank the Alzheimer's Association for the good work they do and information they provide caregivers and families of those with Alzheimer's disease.

# Trademarks

All terms mentioned in this book that are known to be or are suspected of being trademarks or service marks have been appropriately capitalized. Alpha Books and Pearson Education cannot attest to the accuracy of this information. Use of a term in this book should not be regarded as affecting the validity of any trademark or service mark.

# 1

# *What Is Alzheimer's?*

Alzheimer's disease—it's frightening to think about. We've all heard of it. It hits 1 in 10 people over 65. Nearly half of those over 85 have it. Approximately four million Americans currently have Alzheimer's disease (AD), and it is estimated that 14 million Americans will have the disease by the middle of this century unless a cure or vaccine for it is found. It hits people of all classes, ethnicities, and races. Brilliant or famous people are not immune. Winston Churchill had it. Painters Norman Rockwell and Willem de Kooning had it. Actress Rita Hayworth had it. Boxer Sugar Ray Robinson had it. Ronald Reagan has it now.

It's frightening to suspect that you or someone you love might be in the early stage of the disease. And it's devastating to be told that you, your spouse, or parent does indeed have it. But what exactly is Alzheimer's disease? Why does it have that odd name? How is it different from other types of dementia or mental deterioration? Why is it important to be diagnosed early? Is there any hope for a cure? This chapter will give you an overview of the history of this widespread, costly, and merciless disease and a summary of what we know about it now.

## Alois Alzheimer's Discovery

For centuries before the discovery of Alzheimer's disease, from the time of the early Egyptians and the ancient Greeks and Romans, people were aware that chronic forgetfulness and other symptoms of mental deterioration developed in some, but not all, older people. But no one really understood that a disease and not simply the process of aging caused this deterioration.

The actual discovery of Alzheimer's disease occurred in 1906, as a result of the work of Alois Alzheimer, a German neurologist and researcher. Alzheimer was a colleague of Emil Kraepelin, an influential German psychiatrist who had first used the word "dementia" to describe symptoms of age-related mental deterioration. One of Dr. Alzheimer's patients was a 55-year-old woman admitted to a psychiatric hospital in Frankfurt, Germany identified as Auguste D. Her symptoms, which had started at age 51, included increasing confusion, irrational jealousy, loss of memory and, finally, the complete inability to take care of herself. Alzheimer described some of her behavior in a paper: "When the doctor showed her some objects, she first gave the right name for each, but immediately afterward she had already forgotten everything." He followed her case until her death and then performed an autopsy on her brain.

## The Puzzling and Peculiar Formations

Alzheimer used a new silver staining technique developed by Franz Nissl, another famous German researcher and a colleague of Alzheimer's when he performed the autopsy on Auguste D.'s brain. With the new technique, Alzheimer was able to see that many of her brain cells had totally disappeared, which was unusual for someone so young. Then he made two startling new discoveries. He wrote in his report on the case, "Inside an apparently normal-looking (nerve) cell, one or more single fibers could be observed that became prominent through their striking thickness. At a more advanced stage ... they accumulated, forming dense bundles." He named these dense bundles, which looked like twisted knots of rope, neurofibrillary tangles.

Then he noticed something else: "Dispersed over the entire cortex, and in large numbers, [were] peculiar formations." These formations were different from the tangles he had first noticed. They were circular structures, that were outside of nerve cells and embedded in the brain tissue. These spheres also had many irregularly shaped neural structures surrounding them, which appeared to be patches of degenerating parts of nerve cells. Alzheimer named these formations senile plaques. They are now referred to as neuritic plaques or amyloid plaques.

## Alzheimer Reveals His Findings

Alzheimer first presented his research before a meeting of psychiatrists in Germany in 1906. Then, in a medical journal article published the following year, he speculated that the nerve tangles and plaques were responsible for Auguste D.'s dementia. He wrote, "On the whole, it is evident that we are dealing with a peculiar, little-known disease process." During the next 5 years, 12 other cases of this new disease were reported. In 1910, Emil Kraepelin, Alzheimer's mentor, proposed naming the disease after Dr. Alzheimer, which is why it is called Alzheimer's disease today. The presence of the tangles and plaques, which Alzheimer discovered in the brain, are still the only way to confirm a probable diagnosis of Alzheimer's disease. For almost 50 years after Alzheimer's discovery, physicians thought that the disease was fairly rare. Today, however, we know that Alzheimer's disease is the most common cause of dementia.

## The Continuing Puzzle of Alzheimer's

It's almost a century later and we still do not know why the nerve damage Dr. Alzheimer described occurs in the brain. The good news is that some issues are becoming clearer as more attention is directed toward AD and more research is done. At the time Alzheimer discovered the disease, it was assumed—because his patient was only 55—that the dementia he described affected people younger than 65 and was fairly rare. When people over 65 experienced mental difficulties, it was still assumed that mental functions just deteriorated with

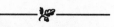

There appears to be a correlation between Alzheimer's disease and strokes. In 1986, scientists began a study with a group of 678 nuns over the age of 75. In one set of results from this ongoing study, 61 of the deceased nuns' brains were autopsied. All of the brains had the typical look of a brain of someone with advanced Alzheimer's. Only 42 of the nuns, however, had been suffering from AD at the time they died. The other 19 had been free of any memory loss or mental deterioration. As scientists tried to find the reason for this, they discovered that the 19 nuns without AD had never had any strokes, whereas most of the nuns with Alzheimer's symptoms had obvious stroke damage in their brains.

age. We now know that Alzheimer's disease can be the cause of dementia that occurs both at a younger age and in older people. We also know that mental deterioration is not an inevitable result of the aging process. It is the result of a disease—either Alzheimer's or one of several others.

## The Types of Alzheimer's

Alzheimer's disease can strike someone as young as 40 or, more often, much older people. If the symptoms of the disease begin before age 60 or 65, it is termed early onset Alzheimer's disease. If the symptoms begin after age 60 or 65, it is termed late-onset Alzheimer's disease.

In addition to categorizing Alzheimer's disease by the age at the onset of symptoms, we now know that in about 5 percent of Alzheimer's cases, there is a family history of the disease. Familial Alzheimer's disease is genetic, so it can be inherited from a parent. This type of Alzheimer's disease, however, represents only a small portion of those affected by AD.

How does a doctor know if a patient's Alzheimer's disease is of the familial type? Generally, if AD can be traced over several generations within a family, and if the family members who have had the disease show a similar age at onset of symptoms and a similar duration of the disease, the physician may suspect that it is familial Alzheimer's.

Will you get AD if a parent or sibling has it? Current research indicates that you have almost double the risk of developing the disease than those without a family history, but that is all we know. One recent study reported that people with both parents affected with Alzheimer's disease had one and a half times the risk of contracting the disease than those people with just one affected parent. Also, those with two affected parents had a five times greater risk than people who didn't have a parent with Alzheimer's. Despite the greater risk, most people with only one affected parent do not develop the disease and, even within the familial type of Alzheimer's, there appear to be other contributing causes for developing the disease.

The most common form of Alzheimer's—called sporadic Alzheimer's disease—does not run in families. It occurs in 95 percent of cases of the disease and almost always has a late onset. Even though it is the most common form of AD, scientists know very little about it, and next to nothing about it's causes.

## What Causes Alzheimer's?

What causes the nerve damage that results in Alzheimer's disease? Even though there has been a great deal of research in recent years, medical science has still not discovered the cause of Alzheimer's.

Some researchers are exploring the possibility that a slow virus causes AD. Others are looking into environmental factors. Aluminum, zinc, and other metals have been found in the brains of people with Alzheimer's, but scientists don't know if they are causes of the disease or if they build up as a result of the disease.

Alzheimer's disease is probably not caused by any single factor, but rather by several factors that affect each person differently. Despite the lack of success in determining a cause for AD, many studies have identified a number of risk factors for

Alzheimer's. These risk factors may combine to increase a person's chance of developing AD. Some of the more widely accepted risk factors include:

- **Increasing age.** Between the ages of 65 and 74, only 3 percent of the population has Alzheimer's. From ages 75 to 84, the percent of people affected increases to about 15 percent. For those age 85 and older, the disease affects almost 50 percent of the population.

- **Family history and genetics.** Researchers have determined that genes on four chromosomes are associated with and seem to increase the risk of AD.

- **Gender.** Women have a somewhat greater risk of contracting AD than men, probably because they generally live longer than men.

- **Ethnicity.** African Americans and Hispanics are two to four times more likely than Caucasians to develop Alzheimer's by age 90. Cherokee Indians, on the other hand, appear to have a decreased risk of contracting the disease. Japanese people living in Japan have a lower risk for the disease than Japanese Americans. Environmental factors and differences in diet probably account for the different risk factors of racial groups.

- **High-fat diet.** Studies have shown that a high-fat diet with lots of meat may increase the risk of Alzheimer's.

- **Cardiovascular disease.** Diseases that damage the blood vessels, including heart disease, stroke, high blood pressure, and diabetes can contribute to the development of Alzheimer's because they reduce the blood flow to the brain.

- **Lack of exercise.** Studies have shown that exercise not only helps prevent cardiovascular disease, it also helps prevent AD.

- **Smoking.** Smokers are at a significantly greater risk of contracting AD than nonsmokers. This is hardly a surprise because smoking also increases the risk for strokes and heart disease.

- **Down syndrome.** Children born with Down syndrome have a high risk of contracting AD in adulthood.

- **Head injuries.** There is a correlation between head traumas and an increased risk of AD.

Again, these risk factors are not causes of the disease. They are only conditions that seem to correlate with a higher incidence of Alzheimer's. Some of them—like age or gender—we can't or wouldn't want to change, so it makes sense to try to improve the areas in which we do have control.

In addition to determining risk factors for the development of AD, new research has identified lifestyle changes, nutrients, and drugs that might help prevent Alzheimer's disease. These potential protective factors include …

- **Exercise.** Exercise helps the heart pump blood everywhere, including to your brain, thus helping protect against brain damage and AD. Since exercise appears to help keep your brain cells healthy as you get older, it's more than smart to exercise regularly.

- **Antioxidants.** Antioxidants are found in fruits and vegetables and in vitamin A, vitamin C, vitamin E, the mineral selenium, and other supplements. They protect against cell-destroying free radicals and thus may help protect you from developing AD.

- **Estrogen.** Women who take estrogen after menopause apparently develop AD less frequently than those who don't. Estrogen, however, does not help those who already have AD and it increases the risk of breast cancer.

- **Nonsteroidal anti-inflammatory drugs.** Who would think that taking an aspirin or ibuprofen for a headache would help prevent Alzheimer's? In fact, people with severe arthritis who take one of these drugs every day have a very low rate of AD. Researchers have discovered that inflammation of brain tissue plays a role in the development of the neurofibrillary tangles and plaques of Alzheimer's disease. Since these drugs have an anti-inflammatory action, they can be helpful in the prevention and even in the treatment of AD.

- **Mental activity.** There is some evidence that keeping an active mind will help prevent AD—sort of a "use it or lose it" school of thought. Nothing is proven, but you might as well use your brain.

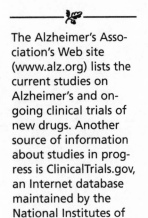

The Alzheimer's Association's Web site (www.alz.org) lists the current studies on Alzheimer's and ongoing clinical trials of new drugs. Another source of information about studies in progress is ClinicalTrials.gov, an Internet database maintained by the National Institutes of Health.

None of these protective factors is guaranteed to prevent Alzheimer's disease. Unfortunately, scientists just don't know yet what causes AD or how to prevent it.

## A Cure in Sight?

There is no cure for Alzheimer's disease. There is no treatment that can reverse the mental deterioration someone with the disease is experiencing. On a hopeful note, however, in very recent years, a few new treatments—both drug treatments and nondrug treatments—have been developed that seem to delay the progression of the disease in some people. There is also promising research being done on a possible vaccine for Alzheimer's disease.

To take advantage of the new treatments available, it is important to get a diagnosis of the disease as early as possible. The various treatment options for Alzheimer's disease will be covered in more detail in later chapters of this book, but the following is an overview of the kind of new treatments that may help delay the progression of the disease or improve the quality of life for both the patient and the caregiver.

Although it is of little consolation to those who are dealing with the disease now, many experts predict that within the next decade, the treatment of Alzheimer's will be significantly improved. It may become a disease that is either preventable or manageable, like diabetes or arthritis. Currently, however, medical science is still in the early stages of developing treatments and there is no universally effective treatment.

### Drugs: New and Old

Four fairly new drugs approved by the U.S. Food and Drug Administration (FDA) help slow the mental decline caused by Alzheimer's in some people. The drugs are Tacrine (brand name Cognex), Donepezil (brand name Aricept), Rivastigmine (brand name Exelon), galantamine hydrobromide (brand name Reminyl). Reminyl was just approved in March 2001. Other new drugs are being tested and developed in new clinical trials that are continually underway.

In addition, new studies have shown that older drugs, originally approved to treat other conditions, also may help slow the progression of Alzheimer's. Drugs in this category include nonsteroidal anti-inflammatory drugs, like aspirin.

## Therapy and Lifestyle Changes

Several psychological therapies have been successful in helping people with AD maintain their ability to function longer. Therapy has also been effective in helping the affected person deal with the depression that he or she is likely to experience after the diagnosis and in the early stage of the disease.

Everyday lifestyle changes can also improve the quality of life for both AD patients and their caregivers and minimize the need for medications with side effects that can hasten mental decline. Some examples include exercise, massage, aromatherapy, music therapy, and even the presence of pets.

Nutrients and supplements have also been shown to slow mental decline. There is particular hope for vitamin E in the treatment of Alzheimer's. In some studies, herbal supplements such as gingko and the amino acid supplement carnitine have been shown to slow mental decline. It's worth staying informed and up-to-date on the latest studies to find treatment options even your doctor might not be aware of that might help slow the progress of the disease.

## How This Book Will Help You

You have probably picked up this book because you are worried that someone you love may have Alzheimer's disease. Initially, this book can help you through the process of finding out whether or not your loved one does have Alzheimer's or whether the symptoms you are noticing might be caused by some other medical condition. With Alzheimer's disease, getting the correct diagnosis can be a very complicated task.

Beyond getting the correct diagnosis, use this book as a knowledgeable best friend who can help you in several ways as you encounter the new experiences that the disease will bring into your life. It will help you understand AD by explaining to you in an easy-to-understand format what we now know about Alzheimer's disease. Without understanding the basics of the disease, you cannot be sure that your loved one is getting the best possible care.

Like some good friends, this book will also give you plenty of advice. Fortunately, the book, unlike many friends, is organized so that you can take the advice you need and ignore what you might not need. One thing that is important to remember is that each person with Alzheimer's is a different individual with his or her own unique and wonderful qualities. Each person will be affected in somewhat different ways by the disease. What has been the experience of some will not necessarily be the experience of everyone. What this book will bring you, however, has been gleaned from the common experiences of many families who have lived through caring for a loved one with Alzheimer's disease.

Finally, like all good friends, this book will introduce you to new friends. It will give you suggested resources on where to find support groups and on ways you can take good care of yourself during the process of caring for your spouse, parent, or partner.

It is you, however, who must remember to reach out and ask for help during this time of your life. Taking care of someone with Alzheimer's can be frustrating, upsetting, and exhausting. Reading this book is a first step in getting help. If you know what to expect and know how others have dealt with similar situations, you can spare yourself some of the pain and frustration. And when you are calmer, happier, and less aggravated, the loved one you are caring for will be, too.

# 2

# *When to Worry: The Ten Warning Signs of Alzheimer's*

—❧—

Alzheimer's disease sneaks up on people. It has what is called an "insidious onset" because there is no one single event—as in something like a stroke or a heart attack—which tells doctors that the symptoms are the result of Alzheimer's. Instead, a number of minor changes may begin to occur in a person's behavior. Mom might start losing her keys on a regular basis. Your spouse or partner might start getting in a number of minor traffic accidents. Dad might not pay the bills on time even though he has always been a stickler for doing so.

Some affected people may just shrug off such events as isolated incidents—nothing for you to be concerned about. Other people may worry about their memory loss and become quite anxious. Still others may actively try to cover up their lapses and be unwilling to admit that a problem is developing. You may have to be the one to insist that your loved one see a doctor for an evaluation. So how do you know when you should start to worry?

Fortunately, a great deal has been learned about the early stages of the disease and the kinds of changes—not just memory loss, but changes in actions, mood, disposition, or thinking—that you might be likely to observe. The Alzheimer's Association has developed a list of ten warning signs that include common symptoms of Alzheimer's disease,

———————— ❧ ————————

How do you know whether it's memory impairment caused by Alzheimer's disease or normal forgetfulness? AD memory loss affects both important and unimportant matters. Normal forgetfulness is usually sporadic and limited to unimportant things. Normal forgetfulness, unlike AD memory problems, does not interfere with daily life except for causing frustration and irritation. And normal forgetfulness can usually be improved by getting more organized, concentrating more, or writing things down; but the memory problems caused by AD cannot be remedied.

some of which also apply to other dementias. Other professionals in the field have adapted the list of warning signs with minor changes. We'll cover the ten basic warning signs in this chapter. They can be used as a guide for you to decide whether or not an evaluation by a doctor is needed.

When considering each of the warning signs of Alzheimer's, remember that there is only a problem if the behavior is both more unusual and more severe than a normal lapse and if these events happen persistently. If you are wondering whether or not you are worrying too much, it might be a good idea to keep a diary listing the dates of the incidents that fit these warning signs. If you find yourself entering things regularly, there probably is a problem.

The subtle onset of Alzheimer's can cause conflict within a family. Often, one person begins to be concerned about a loved one's memory problems. Others, including the affected person, may dismiss those concerns as paranoid or unnecessary. It is natural to deny something so frightening. It is better, however, to be cautious, because an early diagnosis can lead to beneficial treatments. When such conflict occurs, both those who denied it and those who suspected the problem should try to forgive each other.

## Warning Sign Number One: Difficulty with Familiar Tasks

Everyday familiar tasks can become increasingly difficult for people with Alzheimer's disease. Of course most of us, when we are busy, distracted, or stressed, have lapses in dealing with the ordinary stuff of life. We can go to the store and do our shopping but forget one of the main items we wanted. We can make dinner and serve it but, until our dinner companion or our sense of smell reminds us, forget the bread we left to warm in the oven.

With Alzheimer's disease, the difficulty with familiar tasks is more severe. You could go to the store and forget to stop at the checkout counter to pay. You could make the meal, put it on the counter, wander into another room to do something else, and forget that you made the meal. When difficulties with familiar tasks like this occur on a regular basis, it is a cause for concern.

## Warning Sign Number Two: Slipping Job Performance

Because the onset of Alzheimer's disease can occur at a fairly early age, some people who are diagnosed with the disease are still holding down a regular job. Even many retired people who are diagnosed with Alzheimer's may have regular volunteer activities or part-time work with important responsibilities.

Memory loss in the early stages of Alzheimer's disease can adversely affect job skills and the performance of tasks that were previously easily accomplished by the affected person. Frequent memory lapses or confusion at work or in other regular activities may signify a serious problem.

Again, it is important to distinguish between normal problems and those that could be associated with Alzheimer's. Behaviors like forgetting where you left your portable phone or glasses are normal. Walking into a room, forgetting why you went there, and remembering the reason later is also normal. Occasionally forgetting an assignment, deadline, or colleague's name is not a cause for worry.

You should begin to get concerned, however, if you or your loved one experiences these kinds of things regularly and they begin to interfere with daily life or job performance. People with AD forget things much more often and may not remember them later. They often experience unexplainable confusion at home or in the workplace. When this happens, it definitely might warrant a complete medical evaluation.

## Warning Sign Number Three: Language Difficulties

The third warning sign is you or your loved one developing regular problems with language. Again, everyone has occasional

Driving is an example of a complex task of daily life. It requires making split-second decisions and processing a lot of continually changing information—abilities that can begin to be undermined in the early stages of AD. Researchers in Sweden and Finland performed autopsies on 98 individuals aged 65 to 90 who had been killed in auto accidents. Although none of these people had been diagnosed with AD, one third had the changes in their brains that were definitely characteristic of Alzheimer's disease. Another 20 percent had changes in their brain tissue that indicated very early stages of Alzheimer's disease. So, given the complexity of driving, an increasing number of fender-benders or accidents can be a very telling warning sign of Alzheimer's.

trouble finding the right word or remembering a person's name. That alone is not a sign of Alzheimer's. A person with Alzheimer's disease may instead completely forget simple words in a sentence and substitute inappropriate words, making his or her sentences difficult to understand or even incomprehensible. The difference between normal problems and those that might be symptoms of Alzheimer's has to do with the severity or unusual nature of the problem and the fact that it happens regularly.

A common characteristic of Alzheimer's disease is the inability to think of the right word—called anomia. In early stages of the disease, this problem is usually confined to words for things the affected person doesn't come into contact with very often. As the disease progresses, however, even familiar words describing familiar objects are affected. The person recognizes the object—for example, a key, a book, a pair of gloves—but can't think of the name for it. Dr. Alzheimer's original patient, for example, couldn't recall the word for "jug," so she called it a "pourer."

Many people in the early stages of the disease are aware when they can't think of the right word for something. The person may try to make up for it by either substituting a similar word or describing in a long, wordy phrase or sentence the object he or she cannot name. In later stages of AD, as we'll see, the affected person may not even recognize a familiar person or object. This is called agnosia.

In the earliest stages of AD, the affected person's language difficulties may be too subtle to be noticed by other people—even by doctors. As with other symptoms of AD, sometimes a person may be able to conceal his or her problems with language. If you notice, he or she may get irritated and make an excuse for the lapse. Fortunately, problems with language can be detected by neuropsychological tests that might, for example, require the person to list specific words in a group, such as fruits or animals. That is why it is important to take the affected person in for a complete evaluation when you begin to suspect a problem.

## Warning Sign Number Four: Confusion of Time and Place

It's normal to sometimes forget the day of the week or even to momentarily forget where you are. People with Alzheimer's, however, can become lost on their own street. They can suddenly feel completely disoriented, not knowing where they are, how they got there, or how to get back home. When traveling, people with Alzheimer's can become particularly confused. They may not be able to find the way back to the hotel room or find the right gate at an airport.

People with AD don't simply occasionally lose track of time. They can forget what year it is. You can ask a person with Alzheimer's what day it is and they may answer you correctly, but when you ask the date they may give the year as 1966.

## Warning Sign Number Five: Increasingly Poor Judgment

At some point in the early stages of Alzheimer's, the affected person begins to lose normal judgment. This is often the sign that convinces relatives there is a problem. The person may pay the same bill twice, leave the house and forget the child they are supposed to be watching, put a dress on backward, or wear two different shoes. Their behavior is beyond what can be written off as odd or eccentric.

Managing money and finances is a common area in which poor judgment shows up in people in the early stages of Alzheimer's. In addition to having difficulty balancing a checkbook or forgetting to pay bills, an affected person may start buying unnecessary items, make extravagant donations to a charity, or overspend on gifts.

*One Caregiver's Journey*

"While my parents were living in Florida, my father got very sick. He had surgery and recovered. After that, however, he sold their house in Florida and arranged to move here to California where I live.

"He didn't tell me at the time, but later he said that he thought that my mother was having memory problems, and, if he died, there wouldn't be anyone in Florida to look after her. He was over 80 and worried that he didn't have long to live. I have a brother in Connecticut, but daughters are usually the ones who look after their older parents. Besides, who wants to move back to Connecticut after you have been living in Florida? Southern California is more hospitable.

"So, they moved into an apartment in a senior retirement residence here. One day when I visited them, I saw a large piece of white cardboard next to the door. On it, my father had written a list of the things my mother had to do that day. I realized then that she was having memory problems like my aunt and that my father was helping her and covering for her. It was the first time I suspected that my mother might have Alzheimer's disease."

## Warning Sign Number Six: Problems with Abstract Thinking

Managing money and finances require not only good judgment, but also abstract reasoning. People in the early stages of Alzheimer's may lose the ability to do simple addition—like adding up the change in their pocket to pay for an item. They also lose the ability to plan or strategize.

Learning and developing new skills—such as dealing with new computer software—becomes impossible for Alzheimer's patients. Of course, new software can be frustrating for many of us, but we usually can muddle through after a few calls to technical support. Alzheimer's patients, on the other hand, will not only have trouble with new software, they may entirely forget what their computer is used for. Coping with the VCR or television remote controls may become overwhelming. In general, the more complex or abstract the skill is, the more likely it will begin to deteriorate in early stages of the disease. On the other hand, automatic actions, such as eating, walking, or dressing and undressing, may be preserved until later stages of the disease.

Problems with abstract thinking are a common early warning sign of AD. If such behaviors begin to occur in someone you love, it's very important to get him or her in for a medical evaluation.

## Warning Sign Number Seven: Misplacing Objects

The memory impairment in people with early stage Alzheimer's disease causes them to lose and misplace things regularly. Although most of us forget where we put our keys or glasses from time to time, we eventually find them by trying to reconstruct in our minds where we were and where we might have left the lost object. A person with Alzheimer's, however, cannot remember events well enough to reconstruct them.

People in the early stages of AD may also place things in bizarre places—such as putting the toaster in the refrigerator or a purse in the oven. And they won't be able to find the lost item again because of their impaired memory.

In addition to misplacing things, people with early symptoms of Alzheimer's will have difficulty finding items that they have always been able to find in the past. They might look in the refrigerator for cleaning supplies or in the closet for food. Misplacing objects and putting things in unusual places are very common characteristics of people with early Alzheimer's. If you notice this behavior frequently, schedule a trip to the doctor.

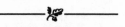

The degree of impairment necessary to interfere with a person's daily activities depends on individual life circumstances. An accountant with her own business will find it increasingly difficult to perform her work and might forget meetings, mix up clients' names, or make mistakes in accounts. Memory impairment won't be evident as early, however, in a woman who has crippling arthritis and depends a great deal on her retired husband to do activities such as shopping and paying the bills.

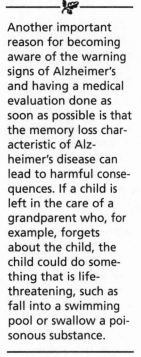

Another important reason for becoming aware of the warning signs of Alzheimer's and having a medical evaluation done as soon as possible is that the memory loss characteristic of Alzheimer's disease can lead to harmful consequences. If a child is left in the care of a grandparent who, for example, forgets about the child, the child could do something that is life-threatening, such as fall into a swimming pool or swallow a poisonous substance.

## Warning Sign Number Eight: Mood and Behavior Fluctuations

It's normal for all of us to have a bad day, feel sad or moody, or complain that we "woke up on the wrong side of the bed." People with Alzheimer's disease, on the other hand, can experience frequent and sudden mood changes. They might be crying one moment and suddenly start laughing hysterically the next. They might become unusually irritated or agitated for no apparent reason. Or they might become uncharacteristically stubborn or resistant to help from others. They might use abusive language that they normally wouldn't. They might spill food on themselves and not notice, or come out of the bathroom half undressed.

One reason for an affected person's mood changes is frustration—he or she does not understand what is happening and why minor tasks that were once easy are now almost impossible. These mood and behavior changes can be very upsetting to family and friends and may prompt them to realize, even if they have been denying other warning signs that the affected person needs to see a doctor.

## Warning Sign Number Nine: Changes in Personality

We all have known older people who seem to become more and more crotchety as they age. Popular movies and TV shows feature grumpy old men or cantankerous old women. In fact, for most of us, our personality may change a bit as we age—as some of our character traits mellow and others get stronger.

With Alzheimer's, however, the personality and disposition changes that occur are dramatic. A person with early symptoms of Alzheimer's who may have been an optimistic, cheerful person might become pessimistic and extremely irritable. A person who was confident and outspoken may become fearful and timid. Many persons affected with AD become suspicious of everyone, including close members of their family. They can develop delusions of persecution. Dr. Alzheimer's original patient became irrationally jealous of her husband. Other personality changes might include increasing self-centeredness, passivity, or agitation.

These changes are usually very disturbing and, as with the other warning signs of the disease, should be taken seriously enough to schedule an appointment for the affected person with the doctor.

## Warning Sign Number Ten: Lack of Initiative

It's normal to get bored with the same old routines. Anybody can tire of the things we have to do all the time—grocery shopping, cooking, business obligations, or social activities.

People in the early stages of Alzheimer's, however, may become extremely passive. It may take constant prompting and encouragement to get them involved in daily activities that they once did energetically. Part of the reason for this is that the disease makes everything so much more difficult. The affected person can easily become discouraged and depressed.

One of the earliest manifestations of Alzheimer's disease can be when an affected person starts losing interest in her appearance. She may forget to comb her hair or continually put on dirty, stained, or torn clothes. Family members might berate or ridicule her for being so sloppy, but a person with AD cannot help these lapses. The behavior, as with the other signs of Alzheimer's, is caused by the disease, not because the person is lazy or careless.

If your loved one begins to lose much of his or her usual get-up-and-go, it is a definite warning sign of Alzheimer's.

*Reprinted with permission from the Alzheimer's Association. For more information call 1-800-272-3900 or visit their Web site at www.alz.org.*

## The Importance of Early Diagnosis

The importance of an early diagnosis of Alzheimer's cannot be over-emphasized. Alzheimer's has an insidious onset and is

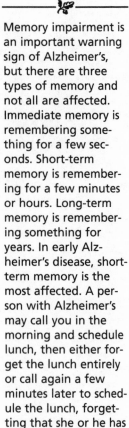

Memory impairment is an important warning sign of Alzheimer's, but there are three types of memory and not all are affected. Immediate memory is remembering something for a few seconds. Short-term memory is remembering for a few minutes or hours. Long-term memory is remembering something for years. In early Alzheimer's disease, short-term memory is the most affected. A person with Alzheimer's may call you in the morning and schedule lunch, then either forget the lunch entirely or call again a few minutes later to schedule the lunch, forgetting that she or he has already done so. Immediate memory may also be affected by the disease, but not as severely or noticeably as short-term memory. Long-term memory, on the other hand, is preserved until later stages of the disease.

slowly progressive. But the symptoms, without diagnosis or any treatment of the disease, may get worse unexpectedly. An affected person may get lost because she does not recognize familiar signs. Not knowing where she is, she might start to panic. When she panics, her judgment becomes worse. Thus confused, she might step out into traffic and get hit by a car.

Since everyone is different, some of the above warning signs may manifest in some people but not in others. It's important to remember also that even though these signs describe Alzheimer's disease, they could also be signs of other medical disorders, of psychological problems caused by depression or stress, or even simply manifestations of normal aging, depending on their severity and persistence.

If any of these problems appear regularly in someone you love, however, it may mean that your loved one is in the beginning stage of Alzheimer's. Because an early diagnosis can mean that the affected person will be eligible for new treatments that can delay the onset of the disease, don't talk yourself into thinking it isn't worth a trip to the doctor. Make an appointment and take the affected person in for a medical evaluation now.

## How Affected People Try to Cope

People in the early stages of Alzheimer's disease are usually aware of their memory loss and develop a variety of ways to cope with the problem. They may make notes or lists to remember things, which may help for a while. They may try to make light of the problem, joking about how if you were this age, you might forget a few things, too. They may blame their problems on others or on being so busy and having so many responsibilities that they can't be expected to remember everything. Because people with AD can retain their basic personalities and social skills for a long time, some may become quite good at hiding their declining abilities. It is natural for people to try to hide or deny these types of memory problems. No one wants to admit that they might have Alzheimer's.

While some people might actively try to hide their lapses from you—which means there may be many more incidents than you are aware of—other people might actually want to talk about what is happening to them. If this is the case with your loved one, it's important to listen to his or her feelings and anxieties carefully. Not only will it be a comfort to the person, it will help you understand better what is going on. Other people in the early stages of Alzheimer's may become frightened and anxious about their memory loss, but may not talk about it. As a result, they may become more and more discouraged and increasingly depressed.

In whatever manner the affected person tries to cope, Alzheimer's will eventually lead to frequent disruptions in his or her daily activities. The problems occur because areas in the brain responsible for memory and other functions are being damaged or destroyed and are losing their connections to other regions of the brain. The affected person is in the grip of a progressive, debilitating disease. You can help by getting them to agree to a complete medical evaluation.

If you are hesitant to call the doctor about someone you love, remember that you know the person better than anyone. Your intuition that something is wrong is probably correct. People in the early stages of Alzheimer's disease may not want to express their worries or may have trouble articulating their feelings. Trust your instinct. It is better to go to the doctor and find out what is wrong than to let the condition—whatever it is—go untreated.

# 3

# Why It's Difficult to Diagnose Alzheimer's

---

Dementia—symptoms of mental deterioration severe enough to interfere with a person's daily functioning—is a growing medical problem. Although dementia can occur at any age, it largely affects people over 75, an age group that is growing faster than any other age group and will continue to grow faster as the baby boomer generation ages. The prevalence of moderate or severe dementia among people over 65 is normally estimated to be about 5 or 10 percent of the population, but some estimates are much higher.

Although Alzheimer's disease causes the majority of cases, dementia can be caused by many conditions other than Alzheimer's. Some of the other causes are more treatable than AD. Others are just as puzzling to medical science as Alzheimer's. We'll cover most of them in this chapter and, while we are at it, learn why it is so difficult to diagnose Alzheimer's disease.

# The Causes of Dementia

Alzheimer's disease is the cause of 50 to 60 percent of dementia cases. The second largest cause of dementia, accounting for about 10 to 20 percent of cases, is multi-infarct disease (MID) or vascular dementia, which is caused by damaged blood vessels in the brain. In many cases, a patient may be suffering from both MID and AD, which is sometimes referred to as mixed dementia. Lewy body dementia—caused by protein deposits found in the brain's cortex called Lewy bodies—is responsible for about 5 to 10 percent of the cases of dementia. Another 5 percent are caused by diseases that only affect a portion of the brain, such as Pick's disease, named after Ludwig Pick, who first discovered the disease. It is characterized by an abnormality in the brain called a Pick body. Parkinson's disease also accounts for approximately 5 percent of dementia cases. The remaining 10 percent of dementia cases are caused by a variety of other medical conditions, some of which are treatable or preventable.

### The Primary Causes of Dementia

| | |
|---|---|
| Alzheimer's disease | 50 to 60 percent |
| Multi-infarct disease (MID) | 10 to 20 percent |
| Lewy body disease | 5 to 10 percent |
| Pick's disease | 5 to 10 percent |
| Parkinson's disease | 5 percent |
| All other causes | 10 percent |

Brain functioning depends on the number of brain cells, how healthy they are, and whether or not there is proper blood flow to the brain to nourish them. Unlike your cupboard, brain cells have nowhere to store food or nutrients, so they depend on the blood to bring them nutrients such as oxygen and glucose. Also, the brain needs the blood to remove waste and toxic substances. Nerve cells cannot function properly when they are underfed or surrounded by waste or toxic substances. Reduced blood flow to the brain is a contributing cause of dementia in many of these diseases.

# Multi-Infarct Disease

Multi-infarct disease or MID (which is also called vascular dementia) is caused by damage to the brain from a series of strokes. Strokes are caused either by blockage of blood vessels to the brain or by a blood vessel in the brain rupturing. Over time, the damage done by small mini-strokes (called TIAs) may also lead to dementia unless treated. TIAs strike suddenly and rarely last more than five minutes. They may cause brief symptoms, such as dizziness, numbness, or a momentary loss of speech or of vision in one eye. Some of these small strokes are not even detectable by the person experiencing them. Others may be dismissed as being caused simply by fatigue. They are serious, however, because they can damage and destroy various areas of the brain. Unless treated, the cumulative brain damage caused by TIAs may lead to MID.

Strokes that cause MID inhibit the normal blood flow to the brain. Brain cells then die because they are deprived of nourishment, rather than because of the abnormal growth of tangles and plaques as in Alzheimer's. The warning signs of MID are slightly different than those of AD and vary depending on which part of the brain is affected. If the cerebral cortex is affected, localized muscular weakness and language difficulties are common symptoms. If the region below the cerebral cortex is affected, apathy and slower mental activity are among the warning signs. In general, people with MID have more difficulty in the areas of planning, sequencing, and verbal abilities such as recognizing words, naming, and repeating than do those with early Alzheimer's.

The symptoms of MID may also be different depending on what areas of the brain are affected by the strokes. Unlike AD, which only affects mental processes initially, symptoms of MID might also include some physical problems, such as partial paralysis or slurred speech. And, unlike the insidious onset of Alzheimer's disease, multi-infarct dementias come on more abruptly and generally progress in noticeable steps. The affected person may get worse suddenly, continue to get worse, then stay about the same for years or even get a little better.

———————— 🦋 ————————

A fairly rare form of blood vessel–related dementia is Binswanger disease. This disease can be identified on an MRI or CT scan, as well as by autopsy. Researchers believe it is caused by high blood pressure. The only treatment currently available is controlling high blood pressure, but it is not certain that lowering blood pressure will, in fact, slow the progression of the disease.

———————————————

People at high risk for MID include those with hypertension, cardiovascular disease, diabetes, or alcoholism, or those who smoke or have a history of previous strokes.

It is important to distinguish this condition from Alzheimer's because with treatment, MID can often be stabilized so that it will not get progressively worse as Alzheimer's disease does. One common treatment for MID is low-dose aspirin, which seems to minimize the decline or even improve mental functioning.

## Lewy Body Dementia

This disease, which was first identified in the 1980s, accounts for 5 to 10 percent of cases of dementia. Some of the symptoms of Lewy body dementia are similar to Alzheimer's disease but, in addition, people with Lewy body disease will usually develop mild shaking symptoms, similar to symptoms of Parkinson's disease. They also may develop stiffness, slow movement, and poor balance.

One reason it is important to distinguish this condition from Alzheimer's disease is because people with Lewy body disease may have adverse reactions to some of the medications that are helpful to those with Alzheimer's.

## Pick's Disease

Pick's disease is frequently mistaken for Alzheimer's, but unlike Alzheimer's, it can be diagnosed through a CT scan and other brain imaging studies. Next to nothing is known about the cause of this disease, partly because it is fairly rare. Many cases are not hereditary, although a previous family history has been established in some cases. Unfortunately, there is no effective treatment for Pick's disease or other diseases with a similar pathology.

The average age at onset of symptoms of Pick's disease is about 58 years. The earliest symptoms may be different from early AD in that they involve the loss of normal inhibitions. The affected person might touch or kiss strangers or engage in sexually inappropriate acts. He or she might wander around without clothes, urinate in inappropriate places, or engage in other impulsive and childlike behaviors. Another common symptom of Pick's disease involves eating or drinking inedible things or chewing on one's own fingers or hands. With AD, if these types of behaviors develop at all it usually isn't until the disease has progressed to a later stage.

## Parkinson's Disease

In addition to Alzheimer's disease, Lewy body dementia, and Pick's disease, other degenerative diseases can cause dementia. One of the most well known of these is Parkinson's disease. Actor Michael J. Fox recently disclosed that he has Parkinson's. The disease causes a progressive degeneration of the part of the brain that controls muscle movement. Common symptoms of Parkinson's are shaking or trembling and balance, speech, and eating difficulties. About one quarter of the people affected with Parkinson's disease also develop dementia. It is unlikely that Parkinson's would be mistaken for Alzheimer's disease because the muscle-related symptoms of Parkinson's usually precede later-stage dementia. The progress of Parkinson's can be slowed with a variety of medications.

# Other Causes of Dementia

In addition to the five most common causes of dementia—led by Alzheimer's disease—there are many other reasons a person might begin to display symptoms of dementia. Some of these conditions may also affect people with AD, making their disease progress faster. Some are more prevalent than others, but all of these conditions must be ruled out as a primary cause of dementia before Alzheimer's can be diagnosed.

## Alcohol and Prescription Drugs

People who have a history of alcoholism appear to be at greater risk of developing dementia than nonalcoholics, although there is no agreement among scientists about whether or not alcohol directly causes dementia. The effects

───────── ❧ ─────────

Lead poisoning can cause dementia in older people, particularly women. Although lead is now banned in paint and gasoline, many older people were exposed to it for years. Lead accumulates in the bone and bone tends to break down after age 50, releasing lead into the bloodstream. If you observe symptoms of dementia, have the affected person's blood tested for lead. If there are high levels, it can be removed with drugs and high doses of vitamin C.

─────────────────────

of alcohol are also greater in older people, as well as thinner people—and many people get thinner as they age. If alcohol is the cause of an affected person's dementia, abstaining from alcohol can bring improvement quickly, although some mental impairment may still remain.

Almost all illegal drugs used regularly are capable of producing dementia. The more likely problem for older people, however, is extensive use of prescription drugs. Prescription medicine used over a long period of time to treat various medical conditions may cause damage to the brain. The more drugs a person takes, the more likely a problem will develop. Diuretics used in the treatment of high blood pressure, for example, may cause an imbalance that can lead to cognitive problems.

Another possible cause for dementia is the effect of taking several kinds of drugs at the same time. Many older people take a number of drugs for different medical conditions. The interaction of those drugs can cause symptoms similar to those of Alzheimer's disease—memory loss, confusion, and emotional outbursts. Also, drinking alcohol with some prescription drugs can lead to symptoms of dementia. Some prescription drugs can also cause depression, which can, in turn, cause symptoms that mimic those of Alzheimer's or other dementias.

## Environmental Toxins

Other common substances to which people are exposed—to a greater or lesser degree—can have a toxic affect on the brain. They include poisons, such as carbon monoxide and various metals and chemicals, which may be in ordinary household cleaning products, paints, or polishes. New carpets, drapes, or furnishings may emit formaldehyde, which can be very harmful to the brain. Older people (and children) are often more sensitive to low-level exposure to these kinds of toxins. Also, older people may spend more time indoors and thus have more exposure to common indoor air pollutants.

## Infections or Viruses

Dementia can be caused by one of several infections that affect the brain. These include late-stage syphilis, tuberculosis, late-stage AIDS, or other fungal, bacterial, or viral infections of the brain, such as meningitis or encephalitis. In the cases of AIDS, TB, or syphilis, the dementias are not usually confused with Alzheimer's because the underlying disease has usually already been diagnosed from symptoms that show up earlier than the dementia, which generally only appears in the later stages of those diseases. In other more rare infections, however, the symptoms could be confused with the symptoms of Alzheimer's and only a complete medical exam could differentiate the infectious disease from Alzheimer's.

Creutzfeldt-Jakob disease and mad cow disease are fairly rare dementing illnesses that appear to be caused by a transmissible infectious agent. In mad cow disease, the infectious agent is found in beef from cows infected with the disease. The symptoms of Creutzfeldt-Jakob get more severe much more rapidly than those of Alzheimer's disease, and it's unlikely that someone with this disease would be misdiagnosed as having Alzheimer's.

## Tumors and Other Structural Disorders

Dementia can be a symptom of injuries, tumors, or other problems that cause structural damage to the brain. Either benign or cancerous brain tumors, depending on where they are located in the brain, can affect mental competency. Head traumas can also cause injuries that may lead to dementia.

Subdural hematomas, sometimes caused by head traumas, are a frequent cause of symptoms of dementia in older people. Symptoms usually include confusion, disorientation, memory problems, headaches, and personality changes. Since surgery can reverse the damage in most cases, it's very important that the affected person see a doctor after any kind of head injury.

Normal-pressure hydrocephalus is another structural disorder that deserves mention, even though it is fairly uncommon. It is characterized by an obstruction in the flow of cerebrospinal fluid, which causes a buildup of this fluid on the brain.

―――――――― ❦ ――――――――

Memory loss, the most common sign of AD, can also be simply a result of living a long life. Doctors call the benign forgetfulness in older people age-associated memory impairment. Memory loss that is severe enough to interfere with routine activities, however, is not normal. There is now a seven-minute screening test developed by Paul Solomon of the Memory Clinic at the Southwestern Vermont Medical Center that can help distinguish between those with normal memory loss and those with Alzheimer's.

――――――――――――――――――

Symptoms of the condition include dementia, urinary incontinence, and difficulty in walking. The condition may be caused by diseases like meningitis or encephalitis, or by head injury. If diagnosed early, normal-pressure hydrocephalus is treatable by surgery in which a shunt is inserted to divert the fluid away from the brain.

## Metabolic Disorders

Dementia can be caused by metabolic diseases, which are diseases that interfere with the body's metabolism. These include diseases of the thyroid, parathyroid, adrenal, or pituitary glands. Liver or kidney dysfunction is also in this category. There are also some rare hereditary metabolic diseases, such as Wilson's disease.

Dehydration, which will throw off the body's metabolism, is a very common metabolic problem, particularly with older people. Also, simple vitamin deficiencies, such as the lack of vitamin $B_{12}$, may affect the metabolism and cause symptoms of dementia.

## Depression, Delirium, and Isolation

Depression may be so severe in some older people that it produces symptoms much like those of people in early stages of Alzheimer's—confusion, difficulty concentrating, and severe mood swings—and these symptoms are sometimes mistaken for Alzheimer's. Also, for people with Alzheimer's or other dementias, depression can make the illness progress faster. Fortunately, depression is usually responsive to treatment, and with successful treatment symptoms can be reversed. If you suspect AD, make sure the affected person is tested for depression.

Another problem that can mimic dementia in older people is delirium, which is a state of temporary but acute mental confusion. However, delirium, unlike most dementias, is characterized by a sudden cognitive impairment, disorientation, or loss of consciousness. It can occur in people who have some of the illnesses we have talked about, such as lung or heart disease, infections, poor nutrition, medication interactions, or other disorders. Emergency treatment of delirium is essential because a serious medical illness such as bacterial meningitis may be the underlying cause.

Many older people live alone and spend much of their time alone. This lack of human interaction can cause them to become forgetful or disoriented, symptoms that might be mistaken for dementia. These symptoms usually clear up when the affected person engages in more social interaction. If someone you love is isolated and alone much of the time and you are worried about dementia, try to arrange for him or her to be with other people regularly and see if it helps.

## Reversible Dementias

Most of the causes of dementia that we've just discussed are more treatable than Alzheimer's disease. The causes of dementia for which there are the most successful treatments, often capable of reversing the condition, are as follows:

- Infections
- Metabolic diseases
- Nutritional disorders
- Multi-infarct and cardiovascular disease
- Prescription drugs
- Alcoholism
- Subdural hematomas and other structural brain damage
- Depression
- Isolation and sensory deprivation

The other causes of dementia do not have treatments that will reverse the condition and cure the patient, but they may, like Alzheimer's, have treatments that—when given early in the course of the disease—can delay the progression to more serious symptoms.

## A Diagnosis of Exclusion

To diagnose Alzheimer's disease, it is necessary to first rule out all of the other potential causes of the symptoms of dementia.

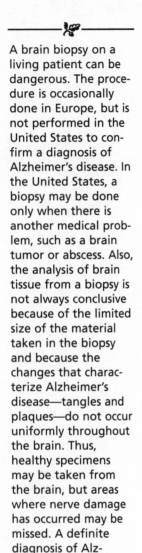

A brain biopsy on a living patient can be dangerous. The procedure is occasionally done in Europe, but is not performed in the United States to confirm a diagnosis of Alzheimer's disease. In the United States, a biopsy may be done only when there is another medical problem, such as a brain tumor or abscess. Also, the analysis of brain tissue from a biopsy is not always conclusive because of the limited size of the material taken in the biopsy and because the changes that characterize Alzheimer's disease—tangles and plaques—do not occur uniformly throughout the brain. Thus, healthy specimens may be taken from the brain, but areas where nerve damage has occurred may be missed. A definite diagnosis of Alzheimer's disease can be established only after the patient has died and a careful study of the brain has been performed.

As you have seen from the possible causes of dementia we have covered in this chapter, there are a lot of things the doctor must look for and exclude as a cause before giving a diagnosis of AD. Some of the causes are treatable and reversible, and those generally will be the things that doctors will look for first.

There is no single medical test that will tell the doctor with complete certainty that someone who is still alive has Alzheimer's disease. All the doctor, and ideally several doctors with different specialties, can do is perform a thorough evaluation. This evaluation will assess the symptoms and rule out other diseases that might be causing them. A number of laboratory tests will be performed to determine which causes could be responsible or which may be eliminated as the cause of the dementia. (We'll cover the diagnosis process in detail in Chapter 4, "The Diagnosis—a Frustrating Ordeal.") When all the testing is done, however, the doctor will still not be able to say with certainty that the affected person has Alzheimer's. The only way to attain certainty is to do an autopsy of the brain after death.

About one third of those individuals who are examined by a physician for memory problems have an illness or problem that can be treated. If no reversible causes of dementia are found, the doctor will next try to discover which one of the nonreversible dementias is present. Only when the medical team cannot find any other basis for an individual's symptoms, and they have eliminated all other possible diagnoses, will they make the diagnosis of Alzheimer's. Thus, Alzheimer's is a diagnosis of exclusion.

The conclusion a doctor reaches is called a clinical diagnosis, which simply means that on the basis of what is already known about others with the same or similar symptoms, and the clinical findings for this individual, this is the most probable condition. It is probably Alzheimer's. Since a great deal rests on this clinical diagnosis, it must be a very thorough process. With increasingly sophisticated means of testing, doctors today are usually able to diagnose Alzheimer's disease with about 90 percent accuracy.

# 4

# *The Diagnosis— a Frustrating Ordeal*

---

Like the brain itself, the diagnosis of Alzheimer's disease is complex. Because so many other conditions have to be ruled out first and a lot of tests need to be run, a number of doctors in different specialties might need to be consulted to find out the answer to the question—is this really Alzheimer's? Perhaps soon, one single test will be available to diagnose the condition, but right now that is not the case. Prepare yourself and your loved one for spending quite a few days going back and forth to doctors' offices or to the hospital for tests. Prepare for the cost, too, since not every test a doctor might want is covered by the more and more limited and cost-conscious health insurance plans today.

Prepare for the ordeal, but don't delay undertaking it. As we learned in the last chapter, over one third of those with memory loss who have an evaluation find out that the cause of their problem is treatable and reversible. What's the first step? Find the right medical team for you.

———— 🦋 ————

Researchers recently performed brain autopsies on 220 people who had been diagnosed as having Alzheimer's disease while living. Their diagnoses were based on the clinical assessments routinely done in diagnosing AD. Upon autopsy, 88 percent had the characteristic brain abnormalities of the disease (neurofibrillary tangles and senile plaques). That is a pretty good record, but given that 12 percent of those in the study diagnosed with Alzheimer's did not have it, there is certainly a need for more accurate and definitive tests.

# Find the Right Doctors

Alzheimer's disease begins slowly, so it often takes a while for family members to realize that there is a problem to be concerned about. When you do realize it, the first task is to find a doctor qualified to diagnose the problem.

If you live in a large metropolitan area, there are probably medical centers in your city that have units that specialize in Alzheimer's disease and other dementias. Often, large teaching hospitals have special dementia units. In some cities, there are "memory clinics" that specialize in diagnosing and treating the causes of memory loss. It is generally best to go to a center that specializes in dementia, memory loss, or Alzheimer's because such a center will have the most up-to-date knowledge on the disease and the latest testing and treatment techniques. If the diagnosis is in fact Alzheimer's, the center may also have clinical trials going on from which the affected person might benefit.

An initial place to check for a referral to one of these centers is the local chapter of the Alzheimer's Association of America. The chapter will give you a list of the diagnostic centers in the area that they consider reputable, but will not recommend one over another. If there are several large centers in your area, how do you decide which one is the best? One place to start is your own family doctor, assuming you trust him or her. Even if it is not your doctor's field, she will usually have an opinion about which center has the best reputation. Sometimes, however, doctors are loyal to their colleagues in their own hospitals, so it might be worth asking more than one doctor for a referral.

If you know other people who have had family members with Alzheimer's, ask them where the diagnostic evaluation was performed or where their loved ones were treated and if they felt the diagnosis was thorough and the care good. If they felt confident in the doctors who treated their loved ones, that is often the best recommendation.

If you live in an area that does not have a major medical center, a place to start might be to call your family doctor to ask for advice, particularly if he or she is someone you trust. Some of the first tests could certainly be done locally, but then your doctor might refer you to the nearest center that specializes in Alzheimer's for other tests. Again, a good resource is the Alzheimer's Association in the closest large city.

A careful, cautious diagnosis is critical. If there is a misdiagnosis, the affected person might not receive treatment for a problem that is reversible. Or, the person might not find out that the problem is Alzheimer's and therefore not begin medications that could delay the progression of the disease.

# The Medical History and Physical Exam

The first step in the diagnosis process is a complete medical history. The doctor should take the medical history not only from the patient, but also from the spouse or someone who knows the patient well. The spouse or another loved one may disclose that the person is forgetting appointments regularly, getting lost in familiar locations, or other significant information that the patient may forget or not want to tell the doctor.

Use these questions as a checklist to prepare for the visit to the doctor's office. If the doctor doesn't ask most of these questions—and more—the evaluation may be too incomplete to be reliable.

- What was the first problem you noticed?
- When did you notice it?
- Once it began, did that problem always occur or did it come and go?
- Did the problem start suddenly or did it come on gradually?
- Have you noticed memory, language, or judgment problems? If so, when did you first notice them, and once they began were they constant or did they come and go?

In 1979, Jerry Stone, a Chicago businessman whose wife had died from Alzheimer's disease, founded the Alzheimer's Association of America. The organization pushes for increased governmental spending for research on Alzheimer's and raises money for Alzheimer's-related research. In addition, chapters organize support groups and provide many educational services to those families who are trying to cope with Alzheimer's. Don't hesitate to call them at any stage of the process.

In the past, when people over 65 displayed the symptoms of dementia, doctors described it as "senile dementia." If the person was under 65, it was called "pre-senile dementia." Today, those terms are no longer used by those in the medical profession who are familiar with Alzheimer's disease. If your doctor uses those terms, be warned that he or she may not be well-informed about AD.

- Have you noticed changes in personality or mood?
- Can the affected person still handle his or her checkbook, do the cooking, or perform other daily activities?
- Can the person work at his or her usual level?
- Can the person play games or do crossword puzzles?
- Does the person get lost or confused in strange places?
- Has there been a change in her walking or gait?
- Has there been any change in the affected person's bladder or bowel habits?
- Does the person have a history of strokes, seizures, head trauma, or thyroid disease?
- Is there a history of depression or other psychiatric illnesses?
- Has the patient had trouble sleeping?
- Has the person experienced problems with weight loss or gain?
- What medications is the person taking, and for what reasons. Does he or she have any reactions to them?
- Does the person have headaches or other pains?
- Is there a history of Alzheimer's or similar memory changes in other relatives?

A complete physical exam should accompany the medical history. The doctor should check the patient's blood pressure and pulse, draw blood for tests to evaluate the patient's nutritional status, check for the possibility of heart and lung problems, liver or kidney disease, or cardiovascular disease. The doctor must do a very thorough physical and explore all possible health problems before assuming the symptoms are a result of Alzheimer's disease.

## Neurological Exam

In a neurological exam, the doctor looks for evidence of previous strokes, Parkinson's disease, hydrocephalus, and other illnesses that impair mental functioning. The exam involves a series of simple tests that evaluate muscle coordination and reveal changes in the functioning of the nerve cells in the brain. Asking the patient to balance with his eyes closed and tapping the patient's knees with a rubber hammer are typical neurological tests. Others might include checking the patient's ability to feel different sensations, such as a pinprick, vibration, or heat or cold in different parts of the body. The exam will also check the person's sense of smell, hearing, and vision.

## One Caregiver's Journey

"After a while, I noticed more things about my mother that made me suspect AD. My mother was a meticulous, fastidious woman. Throughout her life, she carefully examined her clothes when she took them off and never hung them in the closet until she had ascertained that they were spotless. One day I went to visit her, and she was wearing a sweater without a button on it. Another day she had a spot on an item of clothing. It's really important to know how the person lives his or her life. If I walked around with spots on my clothes, it wouldn't be a cause for alarm, it would just be that I was a little careless that day—but not so with my mother. She was never careless about her clothes. So, in addition to the fact that she forgot things frequently, there were dozens and dozens of little things that I noticed that were not in character for her."

The neurological exam may be done by an internist, or as might be the case at larger centers, by a neurologist. If a specialist performs the exam, he or she may repeat some questions in the medical history and even do a short physical examination again. A routine neurological examination will also include tests of mental status and alertness.

The neurological exam will usually be normal if the person is still in the early stages of Alzheimer's disease. Abnormal reflexes only begin to appear as the disease progresses, indicating an increasing degree of brain involvement.

## Lab Tests

A number of standard laboratory tests are necessary for a complete evaluation before a physician can make the diagnosis of Alzheimer's disease. Many of these lab tests will be done at the same time as the medical history and physical exam.

The neurologist may order other tests after the neurological exam.

Blood and urine tests can identify many factors that cause dementia symptoms. If the affected person's calcium level is too high or their vitamin $B_{12}$ is too low, they may exhibit symptoms similar to those of Alzheimer's. The electrolytes in the blood—sodium, potassium, and chloride—should also be checked, since an imbalance can cause symptoms of dementia.

An MRI will show whether or not there is a brain tumor, a stroke, a subdural hematoma, or a number of other possible causes of the symptoms. Unfortunately, because the tests are expensive, the MRI or CT scan may only be ordered if the doctor feels she needs the additional information.

The tests that should be done in most cases are:

- A complete blood count (CBC) to check for vitamin deficiencies, anemia, lead poisoning, and evidence of infection.
- A blood chemistry panel to check the electrolytes.
- A blood chemistry panel to check for liver or kidney failure, thyroid problems, diabetes, and other conditions.
- A urinalysis.
- An MRI or possibly CT scan to look for brain tumors, stroke, and other conditions.
- A SPECT scan (Single Photon Emission Computed Tomography) of the brain.

Other tests that might be necessary in many, but not all circumstances, are:

- Tests for syphilis and HIV.
- A lumbar puncture to obtain cerebrospinal fluid, which can diagnose tuberculosis, meningitis, and encephalitis.
- An electroencephalogram (EEG) to check for Creutzfeldt-Jakob disease.
- An electrocardiogram (ECG).
- A chest x-ray.

Scientists have begun to measure certain biological markers— body components, such as proteins—that are associated with a particular disease. For Alzheimer's disease, tests have recently become available that measure spinal fluid levels of two proteins associated with AD—beta amyloid protein and tau protein. The tau protein is the major protein that makes up the neurofibrillary tangles found in the nerve cells of people with AD. Amyloid is the protein that is deposited in the plaques found in the brains of people with the disease. Experts believe that in the near future, refined versions of these tests may prove very useful. As yet, however, they can't be relied upon to provide an accurate diagnosis of AD.

## Mental Status Test

A very important part of the complete evaluation for symptoms of dementia is a brief, standardized, mental status test. The doctor giving this test should try to put the affected person at ease before administering it, because anxiety can cause the score to be lower. The patient should also have plenty of time to answer the questions. There are several versions of this test that are used. Some of the typical questions that are included in various versions of the mental status test are:

1. Where are you now? (If the initial response is not complete, further clarify with questions such as: What place is this? What is the name of this place? What kind of place is this?)

2. Where is it located? (city, state)

3. What day, month, and year is it?

4. Repeat a five-item test phrase, such as a name and address, and then recall it several minutes later.

5. How old are you? When were you born? Month? Year?

6. Who is the president of the United States?

7. Who was the president before him?

8. Begin with 100 and count backward by sevens.

9. Spell "world" backward.

10. Name familiar objects in the room (such as a pencil or watch).

Magnetic Resonance Imaging (MRI) could become an important tool for characterizing and diagnosing Alzheimer's disease in its very early stages, even before clinical signs appear. A new study by researchers in Boston measured the volume of specific regions of the brain affected early in the disease process. Their results show that MRI might be ultimately able to predict who is at risk for AD and who might benefit from drug treatments that could prevent the disease or slow its progression. At this point, further studies and further refining of the measures need to be done, but this is a hopeful sign.

11. Write a sentence.
12. Copy a design.

A patient with dementia may give wrong answers, say he or she doesn't know the answer, or give an excuse for not knowing the answer. The latter is often the case with patients who are trying to cover up their problems. Someone who is functioning normally might miss one or two of the questions, but a number of wrong answers on the mental status test are a strong indicator of dementia.

In addition to counting the wrong answers on this test, the doctor should also take into consideration the nature of the mistake. A person who misses the day of the week is less likely to have a serious problem than someone who says it is 1966 when it is 2001. Sometimes people function better than their scores on this test indicate, so the test alone should never be substituted for a more complete examination and history. In other cases, the symptoms and history may suggest dementia, but the mental status test indicates no impairment. In this case, the patient should probably undergo further psychological tests.

# Psychiatric and Neuropsychological Exams

A comprehensive psychiatric examination usually complements the neurological evaluation. The main purpose of the psychiatric exam is to rule out mental conditions such as depression. The psychiatrist will usually ask the affected person a carefully planned set of questions that are used not only to discover if there is an underlying mental illness, but to also evaluate the patient's thoughts and feelings on recent events, particularly major life changes such as the death of family and friends, financial problems, or family conflict.

A psychiatric exam is often accompanied by psychological testing. Psychological tests, which are usually administered by a neuropsychologist, evaluate various elements of mental functioning, including memory, language, and other abilities.

They can help identify the type and severity of a possible mental disability and the presence of personality disorders, depression, or other problems that may cause symptoms of dementia or aggravate dementia symptoms caused by other disorders such as Alzheimer's.

A battery of psychological tests can also be particularly helpful in cases in which the diagnosis is questionable or in atypical cases. Patients with high IQs, for example, may do very well on routine mental status tests, but may still be declining in their ability to function. The psychological tests identify more subtle changes in the person's mental functioning than the simple mental status test or even the observations of family and doctors.

It usually takes several hours to administer a complete battery of psychological tests. The information obtained, however, will provide a much more accurate profile of the affected person's mental abilities, which is important in making the diagnosis. The results of testing can also provide essential information for setting up a treatment plan.

## The Possible Results

When the testing is all over, one of the most difficult parts of the whole process begins—waiting for the outcome of the tests and for the final appointment with the doctor to hear the results. Like waiting for a diagnosis that will tell you whether or not you have cancer, the moments, hours or days will pass slowly and fearfully. What the doctor tells you will change your family's life and certainly the life of the affected person. There are several possible results:

- It's not Alzheimer's, but it's something that is treatable.
- It's not Alzheimer's, but it's something that is not treatable.
- It's not Alzheimer's, but it's mild cognitive impairment that may lead to AD.
- It is mostly likely Alzheimer's disease.

## Mild Cognitive Impairment

People who have memory problems but who do not meet the generally accepted clinical criteria for AD are considered to have mild cognitive impairment (MCI), a relatively new diagnostic category. About 40 percent of those who are diagnosed with mild cognitive impairment will develop AD within three years.

Researchers at the Mayo Clinic Alzheimer's Disease Center/Alzheimer's Disease Patient Registry in Rochester, Minnesota, conducted a recent study which showed that mild cognitive impairment is not just normal age-related changes in memory, but is a distinct clinical diagnosis. This study followed healthy older people, people with MCI, and patients with mild AD over a period of time. The people in the study were tested on several different measures of cognitive function. The results showed that the main difference between the healthy study participants and those with MCI was in memory abilities. The MCI participants and the AD patients had similar memory impairments, which were much worse than those of the healthy participants. The AD patients also had other cognitive impairments, in addition to the memory loss. Over time, the mental functioning of individuals with MCI declined more rapidly than that of the healthy participants and more slowly than that of the AD patients.

Some patients diagnosed with MCI will not ultimately develop Alzheimer's; so mild cognitive impairment is therefore composed of two subgroups, only one of which is sure to progress to AD. People with MCI are also eligible for medications that can possibly slow their mental impairment.

## It's Most Likely Alzheimer's Disease

When your doctor tells you that she believes your loved one has Alzheimer's, it means that she has ruled out every other possible cause of the symptoms of dementia and that the loss of functioning your loved one is experiencing is severe enough to interfere with the activities of daily life. It is an agonizing and terrifying diagnosis to hear. If the doctor has been thorough, however, has given all the tests and excluded all the possibilities covered in this and the last chapter, then it is time to accept the diagnosis and move on to the next stage in the journey—learning how to live with the disease.

Usually the doctor will tell the affected person and the family members at the same time. This is generally best for several reasons. First, the person is very likely to be aware that something is quite wrong and may feel like he or she is going crazy. Rather than feeling embarrassed or guilty about the continuing impairment, knowing that she has a disease of the brain may actually bring relief to the person. Second, at this point, particularly if the impairment is only mild, there are many life decisions that will need to be made and the affected person may feel better if allowed to participate in those decisions. Participating may help her feel less depressed. Finally, learning the truth at the same time prevents secrets and other communication barriers between members of the family.

Sometimes families don't want to tell the patient the bad news. Many experts, however, feel that it is best to tell the patient, and most doctors, for reasons of medical ethics and the patient's right to know their diagnosis, will want to do so. Nevertheless, some families still do not want to tell the affected person that he or she has Alzheimer's. If you or other family members feel it is better to keep the diagnosis from the affected person, make sure you have a good reason to do so and that you have considered the possible negative consequences.

If the doctor has given you the diagnosis and you must be the one to tell your spouse or parent that he or she has Alzheimer's disease, it may seem like an overwhelming task. Though there probably isn't any really good way to tell someone he has Alzheimer's, here are a few suggestions:

- Choose a quiet place to talk.
- Choose a time when you and the affected person are both calm.
- Don't try to explain everything at once.
- Answer questions directly and honestly.
- Be prepared to repeat your answers, if necessary.

Although it is now possible to test for a gene that has been linked to late-onset Alzheimer's disease, many people who carry the gene do not go on to develop the disease. Since testing positive doesn't mean you will get AD, it doesn't seem wise for people without symptoms to test for the gene. Getting a positive result will definitely lead to increased worry, and it could also cause problems with health or life insurance.

- Explain that the changes are gradual and his quality of life may not diminish for several years.
- Reassure your loved one that you are in this together and you will be there for him.
- Give the person the time and space to express feelings—verbally and nonverbally.

You've made it through the frustrating and scary ordeal of the getting the diagnosis. Now you and your loved one with Alzheimer's disease must begin to face the bad news and start to cope with the changes the disease will bring.

## One Caregiver's Journey

"After my father died, I took my mother to UCLA to get her evaluated, to see whether it really was AD or whether it might be something else. I knew people often get worse when a spouse dies, but that didn't seem to be happening with my mother. By then, she had become very docile and wasn't at all resistant to going to the doctor. At UCLA, she had to have a brain scan—an MRI. She was afraid of that, but most people are. Then, she saw a psychiatrist who gave her a mental status exam. And, of course, she had a complete physical exam. By process of elimination, because that is the only way they can diagnose Alzheimer's when the person is alive, they decided that she didn't have anything else—she didn't have a stroke, it wasn't her nutrition, she wasn't on a lot of medications, she hadn't had an accident involving her head, there wasn't water on the brain, she wasn't an alcoholic—all these things were eliminated. After that, I felt sure that it was Alzheimer's."

# 5

# *Dealing with the Bad News*

❧

When you hear that someone you love has Alzheimer's disease, no matter how prepared you might think you are, you will be in shock to some degree. But, at the same time, your first concern is likely to be the affected person's reaction to the news. Most of us would expect the patient to be very upset—after all, everything we have always heard about Alzheimer's disease is grim and horrible. Often, however, at the time of diagnosis, the affected person seems less devastated than other family members. AD patients frequently listen to their diagnosis, display little or no emotion, and ask very few questions. Even those who admit to their memory loss and other symptoms ordinarily do not appear overwhelmed by the news.

Why do AD patients often display a calm acceptance in the face of such terrible news? One reason for a more subdued initial reaction is that most people with AD already know that something is not right. The label of Alzheimer's may be anticlimactic, since they've already been experiencing the unrelenting decline in their abilities. The diagnosis may, in fact, be somewhat of a relief. It may eliminate the need to cover up or to try to compensate for their difficulties.

Another possible reason for the subdued response is that the disease itself may be interfering with the ability to understand the seriousness of the situation. It's as though the disease provides a shield that blunts the impact of the bad news on the affected person. As time goes by, however, the implications may sink in further—both for you and for the person with AD. What will the affected person feel and how will he or she react in the aftermath of hearing the news? How will you feel? And what kinds of support systems do you and the patient need to establish right away?

# The Patient's Feelings

Because Alzheimer's disease affects memory and language, it is not as easy for those with the disease to talk or write about their feelings as it might be for those with other illnesses, like cancer. In addition to having somewhat differing symptoms, people with AD also have differing degrees of awareness of or insight into their symptoms. The degree of awareness that a patient has will, in turn, affect how he or she reacts emotionally to the illness. There will be many differences among patients, but the following are some feelings that an Alzheimer's patient might experience after being diagnosed with the disease.

No one is quite sure why some people with AD have a great deal of awareness of the disease and what is happening to them and others have very little. Some experts have speculated that personality plays a role, but it is unlikely that that is the only or even the primary reason for the difference. Recent studies based on brain-imaging techniques have provided a more likely explanation. The studies have shown that the level of awareness of one's disease may be related to how much deterioration has occurred in the frontal lobe of the brain, which controls awareness, insight, and judgment. Ultimately, however, as AD progresses throughout the brain, everyone affected with Alzheimer's will have a diminished awareness of his or her symptoms.

## Acceptance or Denial

Some family members might accept that their loved one has AD and others might be in denial about it. For the patient, however, rather than accepting or being in denial, the issue is being aware of or oblivious to the disease. It is the faulty memory itself, rather than the defense mechanism of denial, that usually leads people with AD to believe and act as though they are disease-free. They may simply forget that they are forgetting things. Or, the affected person may admit that he or she has some memory problems, but dismiss them as nothing unusual for an aging person.

At the other end of the spectrum, some people with AD may be quite aware of their problems and, when diagnosed, feel relieved that their symptoms can be attributed to a disease. Now they can discuss their difficulties openly instead of feeling embarrassed by them. Most people with Alzheimer's disease, however, are somewhere between complete awareness of their problems and complete obliviousness. Part of the reason for this is that the disease itself has an on-again-off-again pattern in the early stages. One day a person may be doing better, and the next day much worse.

Whether or not the person accepts or denies the diagnosis is not something the caregiver and family need to worry about or try to change, because it is not something the person with AD can control. As we'll discuss later, however, it will affect how receptive the person may be to accepting help from you. If an affected person knows she has problems, she may be willing to accept help more readily than if she is largely unaware of her problems.

## One Caregiver's Journey

"My mother never thought there was anything wrong with her memory and she ultimately never knew she had Alzheimer's. I would say to her jokingly, 'Oh mother, your memory is failing.' And she'd say, 'My memory is as good as it ever was.' In her view, she was always perfect. Knowing what they know about the person who has Alzheimer's, I think family members have to decide what to say to them. For the person who has always wanted to know things, whether good or bad, that is the kind of person to talk to about the disease. For the person who has always denied everything and doesn't want to know things, that is probably the kind of person with whom you don't discuss it."

———— ✦ ————

The sense of touch is primary in human beings—it emerged in us long before language. A gentle touch on the arm or face, a hug or a short massage of the shoulders can relax the person with Alzheimer's disease and communicate your love and reassurance a lot better than words, which might be misunderstood or easily forgotten. A gentle touch may also encourage the person who is hesitant to express his or her feelings to do so.

## Shame or Guilt

A person with Alzheimer's disease who is aware that he or she has AD may feel shame or guilt at having the disease. Often, feelings of shame arise when the affected person interacts with people who don't know they have the disease. The person may make verbal blunders or not be able to count out the proper change, and feel embarrassed. They may also feel general shame at having a disease that affects the mind. For many people in this country, there is still a stigma about mental illness, and the affected person may feel that having Alzheimer's is like having a mental illness, even though it is definitely a physical illness. Or, they may simply feel shame or embarrassment that they are ill and not "normal."

An affected person may also feel guilty about the burden that the disease will put on others in the family. This guilt may be greater if they have always been the strong one in the family, but now, because of the disease, they are becoming dependent on others.

## Fear

Although when first diagnosed with the disease an affected person may not seem fearful or terrified, people with AD often experience fears as the impact of the diagnosis sets in. This is true even for those who have rarely seemed afraid in the past. Fear is a natural and logical response to what is happening to AD patients. Abilities that they have always had are slowly slipping away from them. They can't count on themselves anymore. They don't know what they will forget next, and whether it will lead to some serious consequence. As we'll see later, fear may ultimately lead to increasing suspiciousness and paranoia.

If an affected person realizes that he is going to become more and more dependent upon others for help, he may also worry about being abandoned, even by his loving spouse or partner. He may seek reassurance over and over. It is wise to give the person reassurance, rather than to be irritated at his or her repeated requests. The need for reassurance is a natural response to what is happening to a person with Alzheimer's.

## Sadness and Grief

It's also very natural to feel sadness and grief when diagnosed with Alzheimer's disease. People with AD are gradually losing a very essential part of themselves. It's healthy for the person to talk about his or her feelings of loss rather than to hold them in. Not talking about feelings may lead to depression, which can make the AD symptoms worse.

Even though it may be painful to hear how upset your loved one is, try to listen carefully to what he or she has to say. Tell her that you feel sad, too, but also remind her that there is still much in life to enjoy. Without attempting in any way to silence the expression of her sadness or grief, remind her of specific things that you can still do and take pleasure in together.

## Depression

Depression, unlike sadness or grief, is an all-or-nothing state of mind. Unfortunately, depression is also a common psychological reaction to loss. The more the affected person is aware of what is happening, but doesn't express that grief or sadness, the more likely that he or she will become depressed about it.

The symptoms of depression include, among other things, irritability, crying spells, apathy, fatigue, diminished interest in pleasurable activities, and feelings of worthlessness or hopelessness. If you notice that your loved one is depressed, don't hesitate to talk to the doctor about it. Depression can be successfully treated with both therapy and drugs. It is important to treat the depression, because it can make the symptoms of AD worse.

## Frustration and Anger

Some people with Alzheimer's disease might express the frustration they feel at the loss of their abilities through anger. They may lash out at you or others. There is nothing to be gained by reacting in anger. The disease is the cause of the person's anger, not you. Trying to get the person to talk about his or her feelings might help. Telling him you

There are several books written by people with Alzheimer's disease that might be helpful to you and your loved one with the disease. Reading about others and their feelings may help the person with AD get in touch with his or her own feelings. There are also newsletters that are written for family members as well as for those in the early stages of the disease. See Appendix B of this book for a list of helpful reading material.

———— ❧ ————

In the past, many experts compared the progressive dementia of Alzheimer's disease to a person regressing from adulthood to childhood. We now know this is wrong. Even in the later stages of the disease, people with AD continue to be adults and retain parts of their adult awareness, knowledge and personality. They should be treated as adults, not as children, and should be engaged in adult activities that are modified to adapt to the person's remaining abilities.

understand how frustrated he must feel might help. As you'll learn later, there are also ways of alleviating his frustration in the first place.

## Loneliness and Isolation

Many people become uncomfortable around those who have Alzheimer's disease. They don't know how to act or what to expect of the affected person. They may treat him like a child, or they may simply avoid him. In either case, the person with AD often feels alone and abandoned by former friends and even family members. Loneliness and isolation can then lead to depression. If you are the primary caregiver for someone with AD, be aware of how other friends and family are reacting. Try to help them understand that your loved one is still the same person with many of the same needs and feelings, and that he or she still needs their friendship and acceptance.

## Your Feelings

At some time during the days and weeks following the diagnosis of your spouse, parent, or other relative or friend with Alzheimer's disease, you will experience many of these emotions yourself. You will probably feel angry, frustrated, lonely, sad, and frightened, and you may not feel that you have anyone to talk to about what you are feeling—particularly not anyone who understands. It's critical that you do find a place to talk about your feelings, and we'll discuss more about your support systems in the sections that follow. Dealing with your feelings is very important because you will need to be there for the person you love with AD. If you are not in touch with your own feelings, you can't be there for him or her.

It's also important that you begin to develop patience and compassion for the person with AD and for yourself. Until now, you haven't known what was causing the odd behavior of the person you love. Now you know. You know that she will never be as she was before the onset of this disease, and that is heartbreaking. But for many years, particularly if your loved one responds to treatment that delays the progression of the disease, you will be able to enjoy many things together. Your relationship will change, but it will not be over. You will have to be stronger. You will have to take charge of things you haven't taken charge of before. You will have to endure things that are caused by the disease that you wouldn't have imagined before. But because you now know the behaviors are symptoms of a disease and not due to irresponsibility, laziness, or meanness, you can learn to be compassionate and patient.

As you develop more compassion for the person with Alzheimer's, it is equally important not to judge yourself too harshly. You will make mistakes along the way, and say and do things you regret. Forgive yourself and forgive your loved one. He or she cannot help being ill—and you have not yet attained sainthood.

## Medical Support for the Patient

After the diagnosis, it is time to think about arranging for the support systems for both yourself and the patient. Perhaps the first consideration is the medical treatment issues about which you, together with the person with AD, if they are still able to, must make decisions.

### Prescription Drugs

Your doctor may already have given you some advice at the time of diagnosis, but you were probably too upset to really think about what he or she had to say. As we have mentioned before, there are four drugs available that might work for some people in slowing down the progression of Alzheimer's disease. Unfortunately, current drugs on the market seem to benefit only about half of the people who are in the early stages of AD. Because there is no way to predict who might actually benefit from the drugs, everyone who is diagnosed with AD should probably try at least one of the drugs on a trial basis to see if it is effective.

The drugs approved by the FDA for Alzheimer's have been used to replace chemicals that are deficient in the brains of people with AD. They are all in a class known as cholinesterase

When given the diagnosis of AD, it is all too easy to only focus on the negatives, but there are some more positive aspects to remember. AD is gradual, so you will have many years with the person. Most people with AD maintain their sense of humor and emotional sensitivity until late in the disease process, so despite the challenges, there will still be plenty of fun and loving times for you and the affected person to look forward to.

inhibitors. Cholinesterase inhibitors work by delaying or inhibiting the breakdown of a brain chemical called acetyl-choline, which is severely diminished in the brains of those with Alzheimer's. Acetylcholine is a neurotransmitter—a chemical messenger between nerve cells—that seems to play an important role in learning and memory.

### Drugs Approved to Treat Alzheimer's

| Drugs | Brand Name | Manufacturer |
| --- | --- | --- |
| Tacrine | Cognex | Parke-Davis |
| Donepezil | Aricept | Eisai, Inc. |
| Rivastigmine | Exelon | Novartis |
| Galantamine | Reminyl | Janssen Pharmaceutica |

There is evidence that all of these drugs provide slight improvement for a period of many months in memory, language skills, and ability to handle other tasks, such as personal grooming. Cognex was the first to be approved by the FDA. It is used less frequently today because people who take it must have their liver monitored carefully by regular blood tests, since a possible side effect is damage to the liver. Other potential side effects of Cognex include nausea, vomiting, and diarrhea. Aricept is used more widely now, since there is not the danger of liver damage with it. Aricept can also cause nausea, vomiting, and diarrhea in some people at some doses. Exelon and Reminyl, the most recently approved drugs, both have side effects similar to Aricept.

Although the improvements that these drugs bring about in the cases in which they work are not dramatic, people who are benefiting from them are usually very grateful. A problem with the drugs currently available is their high cost. All of them cost about four dollars a day, an expense that may be difficult for many people. Some health insurance plans cover them, but Medicare doesn't. Medicaid does cover the drugs for poor people, and some states have set up programs to help pay for the cost of drugs for near-poor elderly people. Also, the manufacturers have set up assistance programs for which you may be eligible.

## Additional Treatments

In addition to taking prescription drugs, there are other treatments you and the patient should discuss with the doctor. A recent study has shown that people with AD who took a dosage of 2,000 international units of vitamin E per day experienced some beneficial effects. The expected rate of decline was slower in those who took the vitamin E compared to those who took a placebo. Although more research needs to be done, many physicians now recommend that those with AD take high does of vitamin E, since it is potentially beneficial, relatively safe, and inexpensive. It is, however, potentially harmful if combined with blood-thinning drugs.

Other antioxidants, such as gingko biloba extract, folic acid, and vitamin B$_{12}$ may be beneficial, although more research needs to be done to be certain. There are also claims that a natural product called Huperzine A that is derived from a Chinese club-moss plant enhances memory and concentration, but no scientific studies have been done with that herb.

## Clinical Trials

You should also discuss the possibility of your loved one with AD enrolling in one of the many drug trials or other research studies being conducted at different centers around the country. Clinical trials of new drugs are done in three phases over a number of years. It's important to clearly understand the possible risks and benefits—which will be given to you in writing—before agreeing to participate in a clinical trial. The good news is that participation involves no financial costs, and the risk of harm is generally minimal due to the ethical standards and strict protocols that must be followed.

*One Caregiver's Journey*

"Shortly after the diagnosis, I got my mother into a clinical research study at the Veteran's Hospital and UCLA. This was when there was only one drug—Cognex—and they were testing it. There were people in the study who saw some changes as a result of the drug. I remember one woman told me that her husband with Alzheimer's had been a big gardener. He had given up gardening because he was no longer able to, but after he was on Cognex, he started gardening again. It didn't do anything for my mother, however. The drugs only work for less than half the people who take them. My mother did well, however, in the testing that was part of the clinical trial. She was an extremely verbal and articulate woman, so her loss of language and words took a very long time. Fortunately, she also retained her sense of humor for a long time."

## Emotional Support for the Patient

What can family members do to give emotional support to the person with Alzheimer's? First, family members need to simply be there for the person. The presence or absence of caring people may be the most significant factor in determining the quality of life for a person with AD. People with AD still need intimacy and closeness to be happy. They still need to belong to a family or a friendship group and they still need to engage in meaningful activity. It is important to recognize that taking care of physical needs alone is not enough. Just because someone has Alzheimer's does not mean that he will lose his need for intimate, emotional connections with people.

Some patients in the early stages might want to attend a support group of other people with AD where they can obtain advice and information about coping with the disease. Others might enjoy spending time at an adult day care facility. These activities are helpful to some people but can be depressing to others, so you have to be sensitive to the individual and the stage of his or her disease.

It is also a good idea to arrange for relatives and friends to visit or do activities with the affected person on a regular basis. This gives you, the primary caregiver, a little time off and makes the person feel that he or she has other connections to the world. If the person has grandchildren, it can be particularly rewarding for him or her to spend time with the children, as long as it is in a safe environment. Pets can also be very comforting to people with AD.

Meaningful activity is very important to the emotional health of the AD patient. Patients will feel better about themselves if they are allowed to do tasks that they can still accomplish, such as gardening, folding laundry, or other household chores.

Later chapters discuss some of the changes family members need to make in daily household routines and lifestyle. In general, however, it's important to plan regular activities and design a structured program that will both engage and comfort the person with AD.

## Support for You

You are important, too. In fact, you are very important and you must make sure that you stay emotionally and physically healthy. In order to do that, you have to take some routine personal time for yourself—for the things you enjoy doing. If you feel that you have to constantly be with the affected person, you may become resentful and may end up taking out your resentments in subtle ways on the person with AD.

How can you take care of yourself? Try to arrange time off for yourself by having friends and family spend time with the person with AD. As we said above, it's good for the person with AD to feel like he or she is still connected to a larger community. For you, it's critical to get away, even if it's only for a movie or lunch with a friend.

Stay in touch with people by phone even if you can't get out as much. It's important for you to maintain your friendships. It's also important for you to continue to do the things you like to do. You need activities that refresh your mind and

Suddenly life has changed. You are now a "caregiver." You are taking primary responsibility for the care of someone you love who, increasingly, will not be able to care for herself or himself. Don't just fall into this. Be aware that you are taking on a major task. You will need help from others and new knowledge to accomplish this task successfully. Fortunately, there are many sources of help out there for you if you reach out for them.

uplift your spirits just as the person with Alzheimer's does. And don't forget to treat yourself once in a while. Do something nice for yourself, such as buying a new outfit or going to a concert.

Stay physically healthy by exercising, eating right, and getting a good night's sleep. In fact, exercise is something that you and the person with AD can often do together. Take the person with AD on walks with you or to the pool or gym while you have your swim or take an aerobics class. He or she will probably watch and wait patiently.

Finally, you might want to consider joining an Alzheimer's support group. The best place to find out about groups in your area is the local chapter of the Alzheimer's Association. If there is no chapter in your area, try a local hospital or ask your doctor. Support groups for caregivers can bring you new friends, new ideas about how to cope with what is happening, and simply a place to talk about your feelings.

## One Caregiver's Journey

"When I first suspected that my mother had Alzheimer's disease, I was doing internships as part of my training as a therapist. I thought I would do an internship in the Alzheimer's field so I could learn more about it. I went to work as a volunteer in a day care center for people with dementia. It was really helpful in understanding the disease and what was happening to my mother. I think it also helped me to deal with the situation emotionally."

# 6

# *Plans for the Future*

---

In the wake of the diagnosis of Alzheimer's disease, you may feel that you have too much to do to take the time to make financial plans for the future or deal with attorneys and legal documents. You cannot postpone these issues, however. The person with Alzheimer's disease needs and deserves to participate in the important decisions that must be made before the disease disables him or her any further.

It's easy to procrastinate, not only because you are busy, but also because money and the legal issues you must face are not easy things to talk about. The person with AD may feel that he or she can still handle paying the bills or that a simple will is the only legal document needed. You will most likely have to take the lead and insist on making the necessary plans. Don't bury your head in the sand and pretend that Alzheimer's disease will go away. It won't go away and it won't wait for you to get around to making plans for it.

## Financial Plans

The cost of caring for a person with Alzheimer's disease can be staggering. Unfortunately, unless you were lucky enough to have purchased a long-term-care insurance policy before the diagnosis, most of the costs you'll encounter are not covered by health insurance policies. If the affected person is still working at the time of the diagnosis, as is true with most cases of early onset Alzheimer's, the financial difficulties are increased by the premature loss of his or her income. If the person is retired and living on a fixed retirement income, there is often very little money left over for the costs of such things as hiring an in-home care worker, the cost of an adult day care center or eventually the cost of a nursing home—which can average $4,000 a month or more.

Medicare will not provide much help. It covers people over 65 and the disabled of all ages, but only pays for nursing home care for those who are recovering from an ailment or operation and need skilled care. Even then, it only covers the first 100 days. Medicaid, a national program for people with limited financial assets, varies a bit from state to state but, in general, it will pay for nursing home care when the person or couple has depleted their assets—including stocks, bonds, money market funds, and savings accounts. In most states, Medicaid will pay for nursing home care for married people who have less than $80,000 in assets (excluding the value of your home, car, and furniture), but, like Medicare, it will not pay for the costs of taking care of a person with Alzheimer's in the home.

Legally, relatives other than spouses are not responsible for the support of an impaired person, but in most cases, adult children or other relatives usually contribute to the cost of caring for a family member with AD. Sometimes an adult child becomes the primary caregiver for a parent with AD. How much will Alzheimer's disease cost your family, and how are you going to pay for it? Here are some guidelines to help you think about this difficult issue.

## What Will It Cost?

The first step in financial planning is to make a list of potential expenses. First list your current regular monthly expenses, including housing, food, clothes, transportation, recreation, incidentals, and taxes. Next make a list of the additional costs that you can expect to incur because of Alzheimer's. These include:

- Modifications to your home (see Chapter 17, "Securing Your Home").
- Medical costs, such as doctors, visiting nurses, medications, medical supplies and appliances, insurance, and other healthcare-related costs.
- Costs of help for you—people to clean, people to stay with the affected person when you are out, or the cost of adult day care.
- Legal fees to prepare new legal documents (more on this topic later in this chapter).
- Miscellaneous costs, such as easy-to-use clothing or various safety devices.
- Nursing home costs.

The Alzheimer's Association reports the following statistics on the high cost of Alzheimer's disease: The financing of care for Alzheimer's disease—including costs of diagnosis, treatment, nursing home care, informal care and lost wages—is estimated to be more than $80 billion each year. The federal government covers $4.4 billion, and the states another $4.1 billion. Most of the remaining costs are borne by patients and their families. The average cost to a family caring for an AD patient at home is $18,000 per year, and the average annual cost of nursing home care ranges between $24,000 and $36,000 per year.

——— ❦ ———

Money issues can often create conflict within families. Sometimes professional financial planners can help defuse the issues and keep everyone rational. If conflict still emerges, other professionals, such as social workers, psychologists, and counselors, can help individuals and families sort out the emotional issues or mediate the disputes that often arise when money is at stake. When dealing with the crisis of Alzheimer's, it's better to resolve conflicts right away than to allow anger and resentments over money to fester. .

## What Are Your Combined Resources?

What are your family's assets and financial resources? Do you or the affected person have savings accounts, real estate, automobiles, social security benefits, pensions, stocks, certificates of deposit, IRA accounts, savings bonds, mutual funds, money market accounts, or any other sources of income or capital? Don't forget things like life or disability insurance. Some policies waive the premiums if the insured person becomes disabled, which can be a significant savings. Are you or the affected person eligible for any military benefits? Retirement benefits from any past employment? Do you or the affected person have any collections or valuable assets such as gold, jewelry, antiques, art, or other property? List everything.

Now figure out if you have enough combined income and assets to cover the costs of care. If your assets are over about $800,000, then you can probably afford the cost of caring for a spouse or relative with AD without depleting your estate. If your assets are under $80,000, you will be eligible for help from Medicaid as well as the government entitlement programs discussed in the next section. If you are in that vast middle, however, you may have to come up with other ways to finance the years ahead.

## Tax Issues

You may be eligible for tax breaks that can help ease the burden of paying for the extra expenses of caring for someone with AD. You can claim itemized deductions for medical, maintenance, and personal-care services that exceed 7.5 percent of your adjusted gross income. These expenses include the cost of services provided at home by paid workers or expenses incurred at an adult day care center or a residential care facility. It's important to document the need for such services and keep careful records of all payments. Also, you may be eligible for a tax credit for "household and dependent care" if the person with AD resides with you.

How tax laws affect you depends on your situation. It is usually wise to get advice from a tax professional so you get all of the benefits you deserve. You can also call the Internal Revenue Service to get free publications about tax deductions: Medical and Dental Expenses (Publication 502) and Child and Dependent Care Expenses (Publication 503).

## Government Programs

Since most Americans with AD are 65 or older, they are likely to be receiving Social Security retirement benefits based on their own or their spouse's employment history. Someone with AD under the age of 65, however, may qualify for another program administered by Social Security—disability benefits. To qualify for disability benefits, a person must have worked long enough and recently enough to be insured by Social Security.

An application for disability benefits should be filed with the local Social Security Administration office as soon as the affected person is diagnosed with AD. Disability benefits generally start with the sixth full month of disability and continue indefinitely, regardless of age, since AD is considered a permanent disability. For those who don't meet the employment history requirements to qualify for disability benefits, another Social Security program called "Supplemental Security Income" provides monthly benefits to those who meet financial-need requirements.

In a number of states, there are also combined state and federal programs that subsidize home-based care. Eligibility standards for these programs vary from state to state. They are usually designed for those with low incomes and assets as a means of postponing the more expensive nursing home option. They generally pay for services at designated home care agencies and adult day care centers. For further information about state programs and specific community resources, contact the Eldercare Locator Service at 1-800-677-1116 to be directed to local agencies.

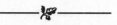

If you suspect that the person with Alzheimer's disease cannot remember what resources he or she has, you may have to play detective yourself to find out. Look in desks, filing cabinets, or wherever papers are kept. Check under the bed, in shoeboxes, under rugs, and wherever you think your loved one could have stashed papers or valuables. You might discover assets you didn't know existed.

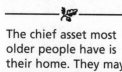

The chief asset most older people have is their home. They may be on a fixed income, but have substantial equity in their home. For some, selling may be a good option, and the good news is that there are tax benefits for doing so. The Taxpayer Relief Act of 1997 offers tax exclusion from the sale of a principal residence for people age 55 or older, for up to $250,000 for single individuals or $500,000 for married taxpayers.

## Other Income Sources

Homeowners, particularly those with low or paid-off mortgages, might consider selling their homes and moving to smaller residences that are less expensive and easier to take care of, such as condominiums. This will usually free up the cash that is now tied up in home equity for use in caring for and supporting the person with AD, as well as the caregiver, who, increasingly, will not be able to work full-time and also take care of the person with AD.

If the person with AD is living alone, he or she might sell his or her home to move in with an adult child. If not, full-time paid help will eventually be needed to take care of the person with AD, and ways to finance those costs must be available.

Another means of paying for long-term care that has been used successfully by people with AD is a "reverse mortgage," which enables homeowners to convert home equity into cash while retaining home ownership. A reverse mortgage is essentially a tax-free loan that can be used for any purpose. Similar to a standard mortgage, except in reverse, it can be paid to you in monthly installments, in one lump sum, or on a line-of-credit basis over many years. Your home's value, your age, and the current interest rates determine the total amount of the loan. The older you are, the larger the monthly checks or lump sum, since your life expectancy is shorter. You are not required to pay back the loan advances or interest until the term of the loan is finished. In most reverse mortgages, no repayment is due until you die, sell your home, or permanently move away.

Reverse mortgages are generally considered safe. Payments are guaranteed by the Federal National Mortgage Association (Fannie Mae), and the loan is insured by the Federal Housing Administration (FHA). Also, before you can apply for a reverse mortgage, you must meet with an independent, third-party counseling service to ensure that this idea is appropriate for you.

# Legal Plans

Certain legal tools should be in place before the person with AD is no longer competent to make financial and legal decisions. Even though it might seem premature, you should make several legal decisions and have legal papers drawn up as soon as possible. Waiting even a short time means risking the possibility that the person with AD will no longer have the capacity to be involved in the planning.

When legal documents are not in place before the person with AD becomes incapacitated, the caregiver or family must petition a probate court for guardianship or conservatorship. A judge will determine if the person with AD is incapacitated and appoint someone to act on his or her behalf—possibly a bank if there is a dispute among family members. Conservatorship can be a lengthy, divisive, and expensive process, but can be avoided if legal papers are drawn up early.

Although it is important to discuss legal issues with the person with AD, it is better not to start the discussion by implying that he or she is about to be incapacitated in the very near future. That will only upset the person, and it might cause resistance. In fact—and you can convey this to the affected person—planning of this kind is beneficial for everyone, because anyone could become incapacitated at any time, for a number of reasons. Also, be sure to emphasize that planning now gives the person with AD the opportunity to make decisions, rather than have others make all decisions for him or her later.

It's critically important to have legal safeguards in place early on. Without them, people can take advantage of the person with AD. Financial abuse of the elderly is a growing problem. People with AD who live alone may be especially vulnerable. Also, legal safeguards protect you, the caregiver. Everything you are doing to help the person with AD can be challenged if there are no legal documents giving you authority to act on behalf of the affected person.

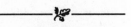

For information about counseling services and lending institutions that deal with reverse mortgages, contact the Housing Counseling Clearinghouse at 1-888-466-3487 or the National Center for Home Equity Conversion at 612-953-4474. To obtain a free copy of the reverse mortgage consumer guide, *Home Made Money,* plus other helpful materials, call the American Association of Retired Persons at 202-434-6042.

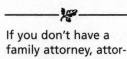

If you don't have a family attorney, attorneys who specialize in the growing field of "elder law" might be a place to start. Ask the local Alzheimer's Association for a referral or ask people you have met in Alzheimer's support groups. The National Academy of Elder Law Attorneys, at 520-881-4005, also provides referrals to their members. Free information on legal issues can also be obtained from the National Senior Citizens Law Center, at 202-887-5280, a public-interest law firm.

## Durable Power of Attorney

One of the most useful legal tools available to families affected by AD is the Durable Power of Attorney (DPA), a document which establishes a legal relationship between the person with Alzheimer's (the "principal") and someone of his or her choosing (an "agent") to serve as a substitute decision-maker. There are two kinds of DPAs—one for healthcare decisions and another for financial affairs. Both are important. The DPA also provides for a second person as a backup if the first agent is unwilling or unable to carry out his or her duties.

The DPA for healthcare names an agent for all health-related decisions and includes directions regarding life-sustaining treatments. People have varying opinions about using technology to artificially prolong life, and the healthcare DPA directs the agent to carry out the affected person's wishes in that regard. Legal forms that provide the general terms of this kind of agreement are usually available in office supply stores, but specific terms vary from state to state. In some states, such as California, a legal document called an "Advance Health Care Directive" has replaced the DPA for healthcare, although the DPA is still valid. It's not necessary to have this type of DPA or an Advance Health Care Directive prepared by an attorney, but consultation with an attorney may be a good idea nevertheless, since you may have questions or special needs.

The holder of a DPA for healthcare or an Advance Health Care Directive has the legal obligation to follow the wishes of the patient as written in the document. Difficulties could arise if the patient will not agree to ever be put into a nursing home. If at some point the patient is not manageable at home, you will then not be able to place him or her in an institution. So discuss these issues carefully before drawing up the DPA or Advance Health Care Directive.

The second type of DPA gives a designated agent control over the management of the affected person's personal property and finances. This document is critical for the future care of someone with AD, since it specifies who is to be responsible for using an individual's income and assets to pay for any future costs of care. Although legal forms are also available for this type of DPA, it is wise to consult an attorney for this more complex document.

## Living Trust

A revocable living trust is another legal tool that may be useful for families with a person with AD. A trust consists of a written agreement whereby a person (the "grantor") gives another person or a bank (the "trustee") the power to control his or her income and assets according to prescribed conditions. The trust agreement includes specific directions about how, for example, to provide for the care of the person with AD. It also stipulates how funds are to be distributed after death and thus can be a useful means of avoiding probate. Co-trustees and successor trustees can also be named in living trusts. Wealthy people routinely use trusts for many reasons, including a reduction in estate taxes, but trusts can also be appropriate for small estates as well. Although a living trust has many advantages over the DPA, it is more complex and thus more expensive to prepare. Consult an attorney to find out which legal tools best suit your situation.

## Medical and Nursing Care Plans

In deciding on the language in the Durable Power of Attorney for healthcare or Advance Health Care Directive, you will have to discuss many of the issues concerning future medical care, including the time when you may have to put the person with AD into a nursing home because you can no longer care for him or her properly.

Unfortunately, caregivers and AD patients alike often see nursing care as a terrible and tragic option, rather than a transition to the best possible care for someone in the late stages of Alzheimer's disease. We will discuss nursing homes more later in this book, but for now it's important that everyone—caregiver, other family members, and patient with AD—agree that a nursing home may, at some time in the future, be necessary and even the best option.

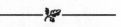

Another legal document you may hear about is a living will. A DPA for healthcare or Advance Health Care Directive is generally superior to a living will because a living will only pertains to end-of-life decisions and not to all healthcare decisions after the person is incapacitated.

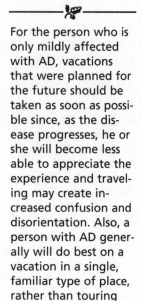

For the person who is only mildly affected with AD, vacations that were planned for the future should be taken as soon as possible since, as the disease progresses, he or she will become less able to appreciate the experience and traveling may create increased confusion and disorientation. Also, a person with AD generally will do best on a vacation in a single, familiar type of place, rather than touring unfamiliar places.

## Spiritual and Emotional Plans

When thinking about the future, financial and legal issues, although critically important, are not the only issues to consider. AD is a progressive disease. It will only get worse. Right now, in the early stages of the disease, patients can still recognize their family and friends and engage in many activities that they enjoy. It might be important to plan now, while the patient is still fairly capable, to get together with children or friends who live far away. Create memories for loved ones of the way the person with AD is now, before further mental deterioration sets in.

It also might be worth the investment to get a video camera, if you don't already have one, or at least an audiotape recorder. Not only can you videotape or audiotape reunions with friends or children, but at times when the person with AD is feeling particularly clear, you can tape "letters" to relatives and friends. The video or audio letters will be cherished by those who receive them—and making them can be enjoyable for the person with Alzheimer's.

# 7

# *What to Expect in Stage 1*

———————— ❧ ————————

The average course of Alzheimer's disease is 8 to 9 years from the time symptoms begin for those who first show symptoms after age 65 and 10 to 11 years for those with an earlier onset of symptoms. Some patients, however, will survive up to 20 years. During the course of the disease, patients will progressively get worse and move through different stages of the disease. The first stage generally lasts from one to four years.

Classifying Alzheimer's into stages provides a framework for understanding the disease, even though the classification is somewhat arbitrary and there is a great deal of overlap among the various stages. Experts don't necessarily agree that the disease should be divided into three stages—some would suggest four, others five or seven stages. In this book, we will use the most common three-stage division, because in it, the symptoms and the needs of the patient in each stage are more distinct.

It's important to remember, as you read about the behaviors of each stage of Alzheimer's, that the signs and symptoms of AD vary from person to person and not every person with the disease will experience the same symptoms in the same order. People will also have good days and bad days, and good and bad moments within a single day. That being said, following are some common symptoms of Stage 1 Alzheimer's disease.

*One Caregiver's Journey*

"In the early stage of the disease, my mother used to do strange things. She went to see her podiatrist one day. She was in the elevator in his building and a friend of mine happened to be in the elevator with her. A strange woman in the elevator admired the pin my mother was wearing. My mother said, 'Oh, do you like it? Here, you can have it.' And she gave it to her. If my friend hadn't told me I would have never known about that. The podiatrist later told me, 'You know, I would make an appointment with your mother and she would never come in, and then she would just come in any old time.' He never knew when my mother would walk into his office. This was before I was really taking charge. She'd tell me she had an appointment, and I didn't pay any attention. At some point, however, the adult child has to say, 'I'm going to be in charge now.'"

## Difficulty with Routine Tasks

Chapter 2, "When to Worry: The Ten Warning Signs of Alzheimer's," covers the warning signs of Alzheimer's disease and the gradual changes in three areas that characterize it: mental functioning, mood and personality, and certain routine tasks or activities of daily living (ADLs). One of the most distressing problems—for both the person with AD and family members—is the person's increasing difficulty with routine tasks that were once easily accomplished.

## When to Stop Driving

Driving is a very complex activity. It requires quick reactions and split-second decisions, both of which can be impaired in people in the early stages of AD. Alzheimer's patients can also become easily distracted by different stimuli while driving. Something on the side of the road can catch an affected person's attention and he or she might not notice a nearby car or a changing traffic light. Common driving problems include getting lost and failing to stop for traffic lights or stop signs.

Driving, however, is also a powerful symbol of independence, something that a person with AD may be very reluctant to give up. In the early stage of AD, the person may appear relatively normal in many ways, and they may not have difficulty driving to the local mall or to the home of a friend or relative. When should an affected person stop driving and how can you get them to stop if they don't want to?

In some states, a doctor must report any diagnosis of AD to the health department. Typically, the health department will then report it to the department of motor vehicles, which might revoke the person's driver's license within a relatively short period of time. To learn the regulations in your state, call the local chapter of the Alzheimer's Association or the state department of motor vehicles.

When the state doesn't take charge, you might have to. It's better to stop the person from driving than to allow him or her to drive and possibly get into an accident. You can start by discouraging the person from driving on specific occasions that arise. Make excuses for why you should drive—say that the person with AD seems too tired, the weather is too bad, or you're taking a new route. Eventually, the person may just let you drive without complaint.

If the person with AD remains resistant to stopping driving, you can ask his or her doctor to help. The doctor might tell the person with AD that they can't drive or write a letter or prescription that says the person must not drive. You can also get your insurance agent to write a letter saying that the person with AD will no longer be eligible for insurance coverage.

If all else fails, you might need to take drastic measures. You can take away the keys to the car and give the person a set of keys that look like the old set but won't start the car. A mechanic can install a "kill wire" that will prevent the car from starting unless a hidden switch is thrown. You can also hide the car by parking it on the next block or in a neighbor's garage. If none of those things work, sell the car and rely on taxis or public transportation for a while.

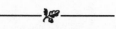

The National Institute of Aging and John Hopkins University conducted recent studies on Alzheimer's disease and driving, each concluding that people with AD should not be driving. In the Hopkins study, more than 40 percent of the drivers with AD were in accidents, 44 percent got lost regularly, and 75 percent routinely drove below the speed limit. It's clearly dangerous for both the patient and for others on the road when people with AD continue to drive after their diagnosis.

In almost all cases, driving is too dangerous to allow the person with AD to continue, even in the early stage of the disease. If the person doesn't understand or refuses to stop, don't argue with them or try to explain—just be firm about it.

*One Caregiver's Journey*

"My mother could drive, but my father did all the driving when he was alive. After he died, she didn't really have to drive. She could walk to places or I could pick her up and take her places. She was a good walker and walked a lot. One day she was taking a walk and went to somebody's house a couple of blocks away. She thought she lived there and wouldn't leave. The people called the police. I'm sure it wasn't the first case like this that the police had gotten. They figured that she lived in the nearby senior residence and took her back there."

## When to Stop Working

For most of us, work is a key part of personal identity. It helps us feel that we are valuable members of society. Adjusting to retirement can be difficult, even for people who retire voluntarily. When a person is forced to leave his or her job prematurely because of Alzheimer's disease, however, the adjustment can be even more painful and distressing.

How soon must a person with Alzheimer's stop working? By the time the person is diagnosed, he or she has probably already been having some difficulties at work. The degree of difficulty depends on the kind of job, how demanding it is, and what kinds of skills he or she must use at work. Whether or not to continue may depend on issues of how safe the work is and how competent the person remains at doing the job. Of course, it also depends on how willing the employer is to keep him or her on.

Some people with AD might be able to continue to work on a part-time basis. Others might be told by their employer that they have to retire. Sometimes those who must leave their jobs will be able to find other places where they can use their skills for a while. Some places of employment—such as law firms and universities—have allowed senior employees with AD to maintain their office for a period of time, so they have a place to come even though they are not really able to keep up with the work they were once doing.

Obviously, when to stop working, unlike when to stop driving, is a decision that will depend on the different situations of individuals with Alzheimer's. As a caregiver, the important thing for you to remember is that it is likely to be a difficult and painful transition for the person with AD. He or she will need your love and support, as well as your suggestions for how to spend increased leisure time in productive ways.

## What to Wear

If you think you have difficulty deciding what to wear, the task is far more frustrating for a person with AD. Getting dressed requires remembering a number of steps, and memory loss can easily interfere with the task. It's more complex than we realize because we've been doing it every day for a very long time. Even in the early stages of Alzheimer's, the disease can make the act of getting dressed frustrating and confusing.

Part of what becomes difficult for the person with AD is the number of clothing choices he or she must make each day. Especially for those with a large wardrobe, the choice of what to wear may seem overwhelming. The person may no longer be able to coordinate colors or easily figure out what is the front and what is the back of a piece of clothing. Accessories like belts, scarves, ties, and jewelry also add to the confusion.

If you notice that the person with AD is wearing unmatched items or puts clothes on backward, it means she is starting to have difficulty getting dressed. It will help if you narrow down the choices for her by putting away out-of-season or rarely worn clothes. It will also help, in the early stages of the disease, to simply organize the person's clothes into outfits. Labeling dresser drawers with large signs indicating what's in the drawer may also decrease frustration by helping the person find things more easily.

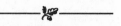

Many people today work in their own businesses. The person with Alzheimer's disease who runs his or her own business will need to decide what should become of the company when he or she can no longer handle the responsibility. Encourage the person to get help right away in planning for this eventuality—from a lawyer, a financial advisor, or other members of the family.

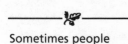

Sometimes people with Alzheimer's want to wear the same outfit day after day. When you suggest that they put on something else, they are insulted and refuse to wear it. If that happens, rather than arguing with the person (even though the outfit may be getting pretty dirty), try buying a couple of outfits just like the one they want to wear. The next day, substitute the new identical outfit and they probably will not notice the difference.

At a certain point, you may have to lay out clothes for the affected person each day in the order in which the person should put them on. You may also have to purchase clothes that are easier for the AD patient to deal with. Buttons and zippers, for example, which can be frustrating to Alzheimer's patients, should probably be replaced by Velcro. Pants and skirts with elastic waistbands are also easier for the person with AD. Slip-on shoes or shoes with Velcro closures are better than those with laces. Reversible shirts and jackets are also great. Pick out colors that always match. If you buy identical socks, the person with AD won't have trouble finding a matching pair. You get the idea—keep it simple.

## Increasing Memory Loss

The gradual short-term memory loss that people in the early stage of Alzheimer's disease experience can affect a number of different daily activities. Their moderate loss of short-term memory might not always be apparent in everyday conversations, but might show up instead in things like forgetting appointments or forgetting telephone numbers and addresses.

To compensate for the memory loss, the affected person may develop elaborate methods of reminding himself of appointments or activities. You might find little reminder notes or lists everywhere as the person becomes more and more obsessed with trying to remember things. The affected person is usually very aware of his memory loss at this stage and very frustrated by it. The coping mechanisms he develops may help for a time.

In this early forgetful stage, you may also notice some subtle changes in the person's conversation, although she seems to be getting along all right in most social situations. The affected person may be more likely to do things like digress from the topic of conversation, rely more often on clichés, ramble on and on, or repeat herself often.

A common manifestation of memory loss due to Alzheimer's is asking the same question over and over again. He or she may have no recollection of having asked the question earlier and thus may be surprised if you respond with irritation or impatience.

At the beginning of this stage, though confused about time, the person still generally knows where familiar places are and who people are. And, as we said earlier, memory loss may fluctuate from day to day or from hour to hour. As the disease progresses to the later part of stage one, two areas in which increasing memory loss will become evident are in misplacing, losing, or hiding things, and in getting lost.

## Losing and Hiding Things

People with Alzheimer's will regularly forget where they put their keys or glasses. That might not seem so abnormal, but in addition, they will put objects in strange places. After cleaning the floor, for example, they might put the cleaning solution in the refrigerator.

Some people in the early stages of AD may begin to hoard, hide, or stash items in odd places—presumably so they won't lose their things. The problem, however, is that they generally forget where they put the items. You may find yourself frustrated because the person with AD has put the car keys somewhere and truly can't remember where. The keys may turn up in the microwave oven or in an old shoebox with a number of other items the person with AD did not want to lose.

Some tips for dealing with the affected person's hiding and hoarding of things include:

- Reduce the clutter in the house so it's easy to find things.
- Limit the number of hiding places by locking some closets or rooms.
- Lock valuable items away so that they cannot be hidden and lost.
- Check wastebaskets before you empty them.
- Check under mattresses, in sofa cushions, in shoes, and in everyone's dresser drawers for lost items.

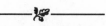

The growing dependency on others to do tasks the affected person could easily do before—especially powerful symbols of independence, such as working, driving, and even dressing—can cause depression in the person with AD. In addition to these psychological causes of depression, depression may also be caused by a reduction of certain chemicals in the brain, including serotonin. Regardless of the cause, if you notice that the person with AD is depressed, talk to the doctor about evaluating the person. There are several medications for depression, one of which might work for your loved one. Since responses to drugs vary from person to person, different drugs may have to be tried before the best one can be found.

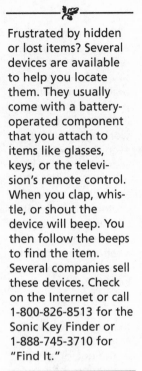

Frustrated by hidden or lost items? Several devices are available to help you locate them. They usually come with a battery-operated component that you attach to items like glasses, keys, or the television's remote control. When you clap, whistle, or shout the device will beep. You then follow the beeps to find the item. Several companies sell these devices. Check on the Internet or call 1-800-826-8513 for the Sonic Key Finder or 1-888-745-3710 for "Find It."

- Make extra sets of keys or buy spare eyeglasses, when possible.
- Make small, easily lost items larger and more visible—for example, attach a large toy or ring to your key ring the way gas stations do with restroom keys.

## Getting Lost and Wandering

Many people in the early stages of Alzheimer's will feel overwhelmed and confused, and start to panic in unfamiliar places. Some people in the early stages of Alzheimer's disease will also start to get lost in familiar places. They may say they are going to the corner store a few blocks away, but come back hours later because they got lost. Getting lost in familiar places is not something that happens to all Alzheimer's patients at this stage. Some people never get lost and others get lost frequently.

When Alzheimer's patients display a tendency to stray or walk away from familiar places and get lost, the behavior is termed wandering. There are several reasons why an Alzheimer's patient might wander or walk away from home or a well-known area. Sometimes the person's medications might be causing side effects that result in confusion and restlessness. Other times the person might be trying to get away from something—like noise, unpleasant people, crowding, or isolation. Some people might become more confused at certain times of the day, such as the middle of the night or early evening. Sometimes the person might be looking for something specific, such as food, drink, the bathroom, or a particular person. Or, the person with AD might simply be restless.

Wandering can be frustrating and irritating for caregivers, but if the person has a safe area to wander around in, it isn't dangerous. Many caregivers overlook wandering behavior until it becomes dangerous to the patient or to others. Or, they permit the person to wander within safe boundaries or follow the individual who is wandering.

Try to minimize wandering by making sure the person with AD moves around and exercises a lot during the day. Provide safe areas for the person to walk around on their own or take the person for a walk as part of your daily routine. Also, be alert to potential dangers for the person with Alzheimer's. Check the environment around your home for possible hazards, such as fences and gates, bodies of water, dense foliage, tunnels, bus stops, steep stairways, high balconies, and streets with heavy traffic. For more ideas on how to keep your home safe, see Chapter 17, "Securing Your Home."

It's also important to reassure the person with AD who wanders often. He or she may feel lost or abandoned. Remind the person that you know how to find him and that he is in the right place. Use humor to increase trust and relieve the tension the person may feel. It's a good idea to inform your neighbors of the person's illness and keep a list of their names and telephone numbers on hand. For 24-hour help in finding a lost person with AD, join the Alzheimer's Association's Safe Return Program.

## Emotional Changes

In the early stages of Alzheimer's disease, the affected person may appear normal to people who do not know him or her. Although the impairment associated with Alzheimer's can radically change the way the person acts in the later stages of the disease, in the early stage the changes in personality are likely to be subtler. Close family and friends, however, know that there has been a change in his or her behavior and personality, as well as intellectual functioning. At this stage, some people with AD still have insight into their condition and may feel like they are going crazy. Other people may refuse to accept the diagnosis and become depressed, irritable, withdrawn, or apathetic.

Some examples of personality changes that might occur to varying degrees are:

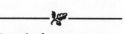

Even before someone begins to wander, it's a good idea to register your loved one with the Alzheimer's Association's Safe Return Program, which helps find and return members home, and the Medic Alert Program, which provides medical information in emergencies. Members of the Safe Return Program receive a bracelet, clothing labels, and wallet cards with their name, ID, and phone numbers. The program provides accessibility to law enforcement agencies and 24-hour guidance to help you find the lost person.

## Personality Changes

| Normal Personality | New Traits That Appear |
| --- | --- |
| Socially active | Socially withdrawn |
| Loving | Self-absorbed |
| Calm, easygoing | Anxious, easily upset |
| Kind, understanding | Selfish, critical |
| Trusting | Paranoid |
| Emotionally controlled | Overly emotional |
| Careful, cautious | Careless, reckless |
| Sexually sensitive | Sexually demanding |
| Friendly | Hostile |
| Honest | Dishonest |
| Flexible | Rigid |

### One Caregiver's Journey

"After Alzheimer's disease started to take its course, my mother became much nicer. My mother was not just a feisty woman, but she could be mean sometimes—and she definitely had a mind of her own. When she fell to Alzheimer's, however, she got easier. This was once it progressed a bit, after my father died. Not everyone's personality changes from what I've heard, and I think it's pretty rare that people get mean or violent."

It's important to realize that these new personality traits may not all develop, nor will behaviors change overnight. The most common emotional changes in people with AD are increasing anger and fear, increasing anxiety, depression, and paranoia.

One common emotional change that may occur in either the early or the moderate stage of AD is increasing numbers of catastrophic reactions to events—emotional responses that are disproportionate to whatever caused the reaction. For example, a person with AD may begin to sob uncontrollably because she cannot tie her shoes. The most common form of catastrophic outburst is crying, although extreme agitation, screaming, combativeness, or temper tantrums might also occur. The best thing you can do about a catastrophic reaction is to first look for the reason it's happening so you can avoid it in the future. There might be too much noise or a situation might be too difficult. Once it's happened, don't argue with her, but try to distract her by bringing up something else.

# Odd and Inappropriate Behavior

In addition to emotional and personality changes that may start to occur in the early stages of AD, the disease can cause very upsetting disruptions in daily life, both for the caregiver and for the person with AD. Certain types of odd or inappropriate behaviors—beyond merely eccentric—are common even in the early stages of the disease. When they do occur, it's important to remember that they happen because of the disease, not because the person with AD is trying to be annoying, difficult, or mean.

## Rummaging Through Things

Some people with AD will obsessively rifle through closets and drawers. They may throw everything out, or attempt to rearrange the things they find. Unfortunately for you, however, they will usually make a huge mess. They also probably won't simply rummage through their own things—they will rummage through your belongings as well.

The only thing you can do about this rummaging behavior is to put locks on drawers that you don't want rummaged. You might also make a drawer and put various miscellaneous items in it that might interest the person with AD—in other words, create a drawer especially for rummaging!

## Stealing and Accusations

People with Alzheimer's disease often become suspicious or paranoid. One person may believe that you are stealing from him or her. Another may make other outrageous indictments, such as accusing you, after you just made a nice meal, of trying to poison him or her. Others might imagine more widespread conspiracies, such as believing the IRS is after them or that someone from the Mafia is trying to kill them.

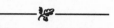

As the person with AD becomes more confused, it is increasingly difficult for him to distinguish between what is real and what isn't. Television and the radio can therefore cause problems. People with AD may interpret events on television as real events happening inside or outside the home. A black-and-white television might, therefore, work better for a person with AD because the images on it don't appear as real as those on a color TV.

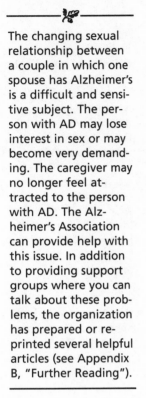

The changing sexual relationship between a couple in which one spouse has Alzheimer's is a difficult and sensitive subject. The person with AD may lose interest in sex or may become very demanding. The caregiver may no longer feel attracted to the person with AD. The Alzheimer's Association can provide help with this issue. In addition to providing support groups where you can talk about these problems, the organization has prepared or reprinted several helpful articles (see Appendix B, "Further Reading").

When the person you love and are taking care of starts accusing you of stealing or other crimes and misdemeanors, it can be very distressing. Again, remember that it is the disease talking, not the person. The mental impairment caused by the disease may be causing him or her to misinterpret information or to have delusions that have no basis in fact.

## Sexual Behavior and Nudity

Inappropriate sexual behavior by people with Alzheimer's disease is not very common, particularly in the early stages of the disease. Occasionally, however, a person with AD might do things like masturbate in public, go out half dressed, or make sexual advances to an inappropriate person. Generally, these behaviors happen because the person forgets where they are or whom they are with.

How do you react when something like that happens? Again, it is important to remember that the reason for the behavior is the disease and nothing else. The person cannot help what they are doing, so it will not accomplish anything if you get angry. The best way to respond is to stay calm and try to distract him or divert his attention to something else. Also, it might help to look for a reason for the behavior. Perhaps the person needs more intimate contact with you or others. Try to reassure the person that you care for him with frequent hugs or other affectionate touches. Just because a person has AD, it doesn't mean that they lose the need for loving physical contact.

# Physical Changes

In general, in the early stage of Alzheimer's, you can expect to see very few physical changes in the affected person. He or she will usually look and feel fine. Some people may begin to experience some muscle weakness or begin to move more slowly. Others may experience a small amount of muscle twitching. In some cases, a person may have problems with vision. They may bump into familiar objects and have difficulty seeing in dim light. They should have their eyes checked. If everything is okay, it may be that their vision is fine but their comprehension of what they are seeing is becoming impaired.

# 8

# General Guidelines for Caring for Alzheimer's Patients

———————————— ❧ ————————————

Although it may seem a daunting and difficult job, you really can provide good care for a person with Alzheimer's disease until the time comes when the person may need the medical or professional care that only a nursing or residential home can provide. You can care for the affected person more easily, however, if you know the basic strategies that have worked for others who have cared for people with Alzheimer's. We'll cover them in detail in this chapter.

All of the guidelines we'll discuss are based on two simple principles: respect and compassion for the person with AD. You can develop respect by focusing on the positive qualities of the individual that remain, not simply the negative consequences of the disease. Compassion can be cultivated by understanding that the disease—and nothing else—is causing the everyday annoyances and problems you encounter. If each morning when you get up you remember to practice respect and compassion that day, you will not only get through the day more easily, you will enjoy more of the time you spend with the person you love and are caring for.

—— ❧ ——

When the person with AD insists that he or she doesn't need help or becomes angry when you offer assistance, it is easy to feel rejected and angry. It's not about you, however. In the early stages, the person's rejection of your help is usually an effort to maintain independence and a sense of self-worth. Later in the disease, the same reaction may mean that the person no longer grasps his or her own needs and problems.

# Cooperate with the Patient's Wishes

It's generally best that you not argue with the person who has Alzheimer's. Why? Most AD patients, particularly in the early stages of the disease, know that something is terribly wrong with them. An affected person might try to correct what is wrong, but the action he takes to correct things may seem strange or annoying to you. If you then come along and tell him what to do, he may get angry and ask to be left alone— he believes he is handling the situation. If you argue with him or try to reason with him, not only will it not help matters, it will very likely make him feel even more frustrated about circumstances over which he has no control.

If you can't reason with the person with AD, then what should you do? Though this may seem hard and will require you to summon up all the patience you have—or develop patience you never imagined you could have—as long as the behavior isn't harmful to anyone, you should simply leave it alone. The best way to manage someone with AD is simply to cooperate with what the person wants when you can.

If the behavior isn't harmful, but bizarre—such as the rummaging behavior—it might be hard to be tolerant. Admittedly, it's tough to stand by patiently while someone is throwing all your things on the floor or repeating the same question over and over, but if the behavior isn't hurting anyone, it's better to let it be. If you are having a hard time being tolerant, try going to an Alzheimer's support group. Others who are going through what you are can help put things in perspective. Or, individual counseling might help you develop the patience you need in these situations.

# Stick to Daily Schedules

People with Alzheimer's disease like routines. They need structure and consistency, which for them is comforting and soothing. Change can be very stressful for a person who is trying to cope with the diminished mental capacity that Alzheimer's disease brings. You can help them immensely by setting regular times for activities during the day and sticking to the schedule.

Regular daily activities—meals, bathing or showering, and exercising—should be scheduled for the same time each day. The time should correspond to the time the person used to do the activity before they were diagnosed. So, if they have always showered in the morning, for example, they should continue to do so.

It's very important that some form of exercise be part of the daily routine. Exercise not only will help keep the person physically healthy, it also may prevent him or her from becoming restless and wandering. In addition, exercise is something that you, the caregiver, need—it will increase your stamina and help you cope with the physical work and stress of caregiving. Exercise is also terrific because it's something that you and the person with AD can do together.

## Plan Meaningful Activities

What else should be on the daily schedule? Providing meaningful activities for a person with AD is not always easy. In the early stages of the disease, the affected person will be able to do many of their former hobbies and daily activities. As the disease progresses, however, certain things may become too difficult. As a caregiver, you may have to find enjoyable activities for the person to substitute for the ones that are becoming too difficult. Since you know the person with AD, you know what types of activities he or she enjoys. Some ideas are presented in the following sections, but the most important guide should be what you know about the person's history. The person will very likely be able to enjoy lifelong hobbies and favorite pastimes, with some modifications, until late in the progression of the disease.

## Music

Listening to music is often very enjoyable for people with Alzheimer's. Music doesn't require a long attention span and it's certainly undemanding. Music can also be pleasurable for the person with AD because it will trigger old memories, particularly when you play the person's favorite songs or CDs or

---
❧
---

People with AD often withdraw from activities unless they are encouraged to engage in them. The person may initially refuse your invitation to do an activity. When that happens, it helps to rephrase the question or simply state that it's time for the activity. For example, instead of asking if the person wants to take a walk, ask if he wants to walk to the park or at the mall, or merely announce that it's time for your walk.

---

music from his or her youth. Depending on the kind of music you play, it also can affect the person's feelings. Upbeat music can help lift spirits, while other types of music can be calming. If you don't want to be bothered by the music or want to listen to something else, it can be just as enjoyable for the person to listen to a portable cassette or CD player through earphones.

People who are able to play a musical instrument may be able to retain their ability to play well into the second stage of Alzheimer's. Encourage them to play regularly.

Finally, dancing to music can be fun and combines the positive effects of music with exercise.

## Gardening

Gardening, in moderation, can be a very healing activity for people with AD, particularly for those who have enjoyed gardening in the past. In the summer, or in some climates year round, the affected person can plant, weed, water, trim and cut back plants, fertilize, rake leaves, or mow the lawn. Just don't give the person so many chores that he or she feels overwhelmed or too tired. In the winter, planting and tending to indoor plants can be great projects for the person with AD.

## Reminiscing

Since long-term memory remains intact longer than short-term memory, many people with Alzheimer's disease enjoy recounting stories from their past to members of their family and friends. In addition to being enjoyable for the person, reminiscing can validate the person's contributions in life and thus increase the patient's self-esteem during this difficult time.

Not all reminiscing has to be done with other people. The affected person can write about his or her life or can make a scrapbook or photo album with memories of his or her life. The person with Alzheimer's might also enjoy sorting through old junk in the attic or basement, because of the memories the things will help evoke. Books from the library with pictures and photos of past eras may also stimulate memories of the past and thus be enjoyable for a person with AD.

Other activities that might evoke long-term memories include visiting certain important places, listening to favorite pieces of music, watching old movies, and watching home movies.

## One Caregiver's Journey

"My mother was a wonderful storyteller. She would tell a story with a very dramatic flair. One day I took my mother to the department store because I had to buy something. At the time, she was telling everybody this story that she made up that she thought was true. She said that her hair turned completely white overnight when my father died. This was not true. Her hair had been white since she let it grow out after being blond.

"So we were in this department store and another customer came in who knew me slightly. She had a mother with Alzheimer's who was going to the Adult Day Care center where I worked. Her mother wasn't in my group so I didn't know her well. I introduced her to my mother and my mother started telling her and the saleslady about her hair turning white overnight. At the end of the story, the other customer said to me, 'It must be nice to have a mother growing old so graciously.'

"She had no idea that my mother had Alzheimer's, because she could tell such a good story and still had good social skills. I just smiled."

## Quiet Time

While you are busy with work or household tasks, it's important to have activities planned to occupy the person with AD. In the early stages of the disease, the person will still initiate many activities on her own, but as the disease progresses you will have to motivate her with ideas and suggestions of what to do.

Reading is a source of pleasure for many people. Unfortunately, if the person with AD enjoys novels, at a certain

———————— ❧ ————————

Books are not only entertaining or a way to pass the time, but some books also can help the person with AD cope with the disease and the future. Many families and people with AD have attributed their ability to cope successfully with the challenges of AD to the greater self-awareness they've gained, at least partially, through reading. Not only books or publications that directly deal with Alzheimer's disease, but other literature may help individuals think about their childhood or examine what is important to them in life. Books can be friends that help people face the loss that they are experiencing as a result of Alzheimer's disease. Check Appendix B, "Further Reading," for some suggestions of books that might be helpful for your loved one.

point in the disease he will not be able to remember the story line. Short stories that can be read at one sitting might be a good alternative. Later, when the person with AD may still be able to read but is having difficulty visually, large-type books and magazines may work better for him. Several magazines, such as *Reader's Digest*, have large-type editions. Also, most libraries have sections of large-type books. Many books are available on tape or on CD and can be listened to with the same portable player the person uses to listen to music. Books with pictures—such as those found in the children's section of the library—can be enjoyable for those in the later stages of the disease.

Television can be enjoyable for some people with AD, even after they can't completely follow the story line or plot of an episode or movie. Others find it frightening. The type of program the person is viewing usually makes a difference. In general, it is best to avoid action-filled programs. Comedy, sports, wildlife, or educational programs are usually best.

The person with AD can also help with certain kinds of household chores. Things like sorting dark and white laundry or folding finished laundry are usually easy enough for the affected person. The person with AD can also help you prepare meals if you give him or her discrete tasks such as chopping a vegetable or snapping peas.

## Children and Pets

Children—both younger ones and teenagers—can often have a very positive effect on people with AD. Children can be very accepting of people with disabilities, and they are often good at getting older people to do things with them—like tossing a ball, dancing, singing or putting together a puzzle. One potential problem with children, however, especially younger children, may be too much noise. People with AD tend to do better in quieter surroundings, so a noisy child or group of children could make the person feel more confused.

People with Alzheimer's disease often respond very well to pets and are usually quite capable of caring for them. Pets offer everyone unconditional love, which can be a source of comfort and delight to people with Alzheimer's disease. If you don't have a pet, perhaps a friend or neighbor has a pet the AD patient can play with regularly—or it might be a good idea to get one. Even if for some reason you can't get a dog or a cat, birds and fish can also provide enjoyment for the AD patient.

## Create a Calm and Stable Environment

One of the most important things you can do in taking care of a person with AD is to reduce the level of stress and make the home environment as calm and stable as possible. Later in this book, we devote a whole chapter (Chapter 17, "Securing Your Home") to ways to improve and make the living quarters secure for the person with AD. Prior to that, however, here are some general guidelines for making the home environment more Alzheimer's-friendly.

First, keep the environment simple. Spare is better than clutter, so get rid of clutter. Too many things in the environment can create confusion for the person with AD and confusion can lead to anxiety or catastrophic reactions. If you don't have time to sort through things and throw them out, then lock the clutter away in the basement or a spare room.

Second, keep rooms as they are. Now is not the time to redecorate, rearrange furniture, or buy new items of furniture. It's particularly important to keep favorite chairs, pictures, and other familiar objects. The only exceptions to this are items of furniture that might be hazardous, such as glass tables with sharp corners.

Third, try to provide information and cues to help the AD patient find his or her way around. Even in the early stages of the disease, a person with AD may become confused in familiar surroundings. You may want to place labels on things such as bathroom doors, as well as to label drawers with the names of items that are in them. Make sure the labels are simple and large enough to be read easily.

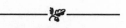

Children generally react to someone with AD as their parents do. If the parents are irritable, the children will be, too. If the parents are patient and explain the disease to the child, the child will usually be fine. Complications can arise when the person with AD lives with a family with children. Caring for the affected person can take attention away from the child, who may react by withdrawing or acting out.

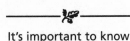

It's important to know what the person with AD can still do and what he or she can no longer do safely. Capabilities change gradually, so make sure you observe the person carefully. For example, Mom may say that she can heat up leftovers for dinner—and she has always been able to do so. Now, however, she may burn herself on the gas stove, or spill liquid on the floor, not notice it, and slip and fall.

Finally, you will have to check the environment for possible safety hazards. Again, this is covered thoroughly later, but in general, make sure that you identify things in the home or yard that the person could either misuse or injure themselves with. Poisonous materials, such as insecticides, cleaning supplies, paint, or gasoline, should be stored in a locked or inaccessible place. The person may forget what these items are for and use them inappropriately. Likewise, keep medications out of reach of the person, who may forget that he or she has already taken the dose for the day.

## *One Caregiver's Journey*

"After my mother's diagnosis, she was still able to live on her own for quite a while. She was living in a senior residence, which was a very structured environment. She had all her meals in a dining room and had maid service, so she didn't have to do much on her own. One night, not long after the diagnosis, we were having dinner at a big affair, and my mother was sitting next to me. I must have turned to talk to the person on the other side of me for a moment. When I looked back, my mother was gone. I got upset and told my husband, who was there, that my mother was gone. I rushed out and was looking all over the lobby and outside the building for her. I was panicking. My husband, meanwhile, got in the elevator and went up to the fifth floor, because my mother lived on the fifth floor of the senior residence. Sure enough, there she was. She had gone up to the fifth floor thinking that she was in her building."

## Establish Good Verbal and Nonverbal Communication

Many of the problems that patients with Alzheimer's disease experience come from their utter frustration at not being able to communicate or interact with people effectively and in a rewarding or meaningful way any more. Caregivers can improve communication with persons with AD and help make life less frustrating for both the caregiver and the patient in several ways. Following are some general tips for establishing good communication:

- Make sure you have the person's attention before speaking.
- Maintain direct eye contact during a conversation.
- Talk in a quiet place away from distractions and noise.
- Use simple words and short, simple sentences.
- Ask questions that can be answered with a simple yes or no, rather than open-ended ones.
- Stay calm and patient, and talk softly and clearly.
- Give the person with AD plenty of time to respond.
- Don't argue or attempt to reason with the person.
- Try different words to say the same thing if he or she doesn't understand at first.
- Make sure your nonverbal communication—or body language—is relaxed.
- Make sure your tone of voice is calm and pleasant.
- Try to demonstrate things visually if your words are not being understood.

People with Alzheimer's disease often become hypersensitive to nonverbal communication. If you are upset, frustrated, anxious, or angry, even if you don't express those feelings verbally, the person with AD will often respond not to what you have said, but to your body language and tone of voice. A slow, relaxed tone, on the other hand, will convey calm and patience. A person with AD will often mirror—mimic or copy—the emotional state of the person with whom he or she is talking. So, if you want the person to stay calm, you will have to stay calm yourself.

Also, your body language, which includes facial expressions and gestures, can be helpful in getting the person with AD to understand you by giving him or her important nonverbal cues. The person may have difficulty completely understanding the words you are saying but can get the point by watching the gestures and expressions you make.

It's also important to remember to speak slowly and in a simple way, which might require some effort on your part. You may be used to talking fast or in a shorthand style that your loved one always understood before, but now has trouble with because of AD. You will have to re-train yourself to slow down and speak as clearly as you can.

A common misunderstanding is that people with Alzheimer's have hearing problems, so people tend to yell when talking to them. This, of course, just increases their frustration. Speaking clearly doesn't necessarily mean speaking louder!

The other important part of communicating with a person with AD is the way in which you listen. The person with AD may need to use a number of words as he or she searches for the right word. You can help by supplying the needed word or phrase, if you know what the person is getting at. It's not necessary for him or her to struggle for the right word. On the other hand, balance is required. Sometimes it's important to allow the person enough time to finish a thought before interrupting. He should not feel rushed and should be encouraged to fully express himself. The actual content of what he is saying may not be as important as the feelings he is trying to express.

People with AD will tend to rely less and less on verbal communication as the disease progresses. You may need to get more comfortable with silences and not assume that it means the person with AD is angry or depressed. Try giving the affected person a hug instead of expressing your feelings verbally and you will probably get a grateful hug in return.

## Stop Blaming

As you realize by now, Alzheimer's disease often brings about a change in roles in the family. For example, if you are a spouse or partner who has let the other person take the lead and make most of the important decisions in your relationship, now, because of the disease, you must take the leadership role. You must make decisions you never had to make before, often without any assistance. If you are the one who has been taken care of, now you must take care of the other person. In any case, you may find yourself responsible for things you have never done before. If you are the child and your parent has always been there for you, now you must be there for your mother or father.

These changes can be very uncomfortable for both you and the person with AD. It will be difficult to adjust to the new roles for both of you. You can be sensitive to her and help her maintain her self-respect by not making a big deal out of everything you are doing and by letting her do as much as she can for as long as possible, even when it might be more efficient for you to simply take over a particular task.

Despite your best efforts, however, and particularly in the early stage of the disease when you are still trying to adjust to everything, these changes may bring about angry moments, tears, and the tendency to blame the person with AD or to blame yourself for the difficult times.

When that happens, try to simply forget about who is to blame in any situation. It is not productive to blame the person with AD, because it is the disease that makes them do the things they do, which then upset or irritate you. Likewise, there is nothing to be gained by blaming yourself. Learning how to accept the changes the disease will bring, learning how to communicate better with the person, and learning how to control your anger or other nonproductive emotions—none of these are easy tasks. Give yourself and the person with AD a break. You are each doing the very best you can in a heartbreakingly sad and difficult situation.

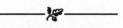

It may take emotional strength and self-confidence you never have felt before to assume the responsibility for taking care of both the person with AD and yourself. The good news is that you are preparing yourself and building your confidence by reading books like this one. The other good news is that you don't need to take over everything all at once. AD develops gradually, and you can get stronger and more confident gradually, too.

# 9

# *How Do You Survive Stage 1?*

❧

Over four million Americans suffer from Alzheimer's disease. More than 70 percent of them live at home and are cared for by family members. About 55 percent of caregivers are spouses, 35 percent are adult children, and the other 10 percent are a mixture of siblings, other relatives, friends, or paid companions. Women are more often primary caregivers—wives, daughters, daughters-in-law, and granddaughters—although many men do take on the responsibility of caring for their spouses or life partners with AD.

Caregivers may have other responsibilities besides the care of the person with Alzheimer's—such as work, family, or furthering their educations. Caregivers who work spend about 40 additional hours a week taking care of the person with AD and those who do not have outside work may spend up to 100 hours a week caring for the affected person.

The additional demands of caring for the AD patient, combined with other responsibilities—particularly for those who live with the person with AD—may cause caregivers to neglect their own needs. They may skip exercising, eat junk food, avoid friends, and not get adequate sleep.

Now that you are among the legions of family caregivers, how can you handle the increased responsibility without the physical and emotional stress of caregiving becoming too much for you? How can you prevent yourself from burning out and becoming a secondary victim of AD? In each situation and at

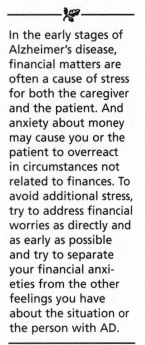

In the early stages of Alzheimer's disease, financial matters are often a cause of stress for both the caregiver and the patient. And anxiety about money may cause you or the patient to overreact in circumstances not related to finances. To avoid additional stress, try to address financial worries as directly and as early as possible and try to separate your financial anxieties from the other feelings you have about the situation or the person with AD.

each stage of the disease, there are different challenges and different strategies for taking care of your own needs. In this chapter, we'll cover some suggestions to help you survive Stage 1.

# When You Are the Patient's Life Partner

In long-term relationships, people make commitments to care for each other "in sickness and in health" and, throughout most successful relationships, each partner usually does his or her share of taking care of the other partner in a health or emotional crisis. When Alzheimer's disease hits, however, the give and take is over. The person with Alzheimer's will need more and more care from his or her partner, and the well partner will no longer be able to count on the person with AD for the same level of physical or emotional support. The expectations on which the relationship has been built for years must change. Now you are solely responsible for your partner, rather than each of you being responsible for the other.

This new foundation for the relationship is a difficult adjustment for both partners, but for you, the caregiver, suddenly the person who has brought you so much comfort, joy, and loving support in the past, will become—not entirely and not all at once, but ultimately—a physical and emotional burden to you. It is hard to face that fact, but it is the reality.

There are practical tips for coping with these changes that we'll discuss a little later in this chapter, but the first step is to accept what is happening to your relationship. Your partner is gradually losing the ability to do many things you have always expected him or her to do. You won't be able to have the same kind of relationship, but you can still enjoy doing together whatever he or she is capable of at the moment. Even with your partner's new limitations, there are opportunities for closeness if you don't expect the same kind of support and commitment from him or her that you once had.

## Prepare for Practical Changes

What are some practical adjustments you can make in your marriage? In the early stage of the disease, you can ask the person with Alzheimer's to help you learn to do the chores and duties that he or she has usually done. If she pays the bills, get her to show you all the records, correspondence, and files before she is unable to do so. If she does most of the cooking, shopping, or housework, get her to teach you some of her favorite recipes, to take you to the store so you can shop together, and to give you some tips on taking care of the house. You'll need them before long.

If she resists and wants to keep doing what she has always done, don't try to stop her. She needs to maintain a feeling of independence as long as possible. It's important, however, that you learn how to do some of the things you will ultimately be responsible for. Without forcing the affected person, indicate your willingness to help out, to learn, and to share the responsibilities. As chores begin to get more difficult for the person, he or she will probably accept your help more graciously.

## Sexuality and Intimacy

You may feel that it's not a priority to think about sex when there are so many other pressing issues that are affecting your life in the early stages of Alzheimer's disease. But sex is important, and you should think about it. You and your partner both still need to be loved and touched. Sex and physical affection are important parts of any long-term relationship.

Your sexual relationship might change, just as other aspects of your relationship with the person with AD are altered by the disease. Alzheimer's may cause changes in your loved one's memory, mood, and behavior that negatively affect your sexual relationship. Each patient is different, however, and it's possible that sex might remain one of the things that you and the affected person will be able to enjoy together for some time. You might even become closer as you struggle together to live with the disease.

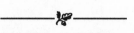

In addition to taking over household duties, you will also need to keep track of everything for both of you. That includes medications, appointments for doctors, dentists, and hairdressers, as well as remembering birthdays and other social events. If you aren't an organized person, now is the time to learn something about time management. You will have to run the household like a very efficient business in which every minute counts.

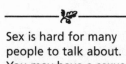

Sex is hard for many people to talk about. You may have a sexual problem that would be greatly helped by talking to a professional counselor, but you might not feel comfortable discussing it. Try not to let feelings of embarrassment about sex stop you from seeking professional help. With the complex changes that Alzheimer's disease brings, medical and psychological help may be particularly valuable in helping you deal with a sexual problem and in alleviating related emotional distress.

What are some of the sexual problems that might occur? First, either you or the affected person may no longer be interested in sex. You may feel too tired or depressed. Or you may feel unable to make love to a person with whom you can no longer really talk to or connect with in the same way. Sometimes the person with AD may also lose interest in sex, particularly if he or she is depressed.

If your sexual relationship does continue, changes may occur that are hard for you to handle. For example, memory loss can cause the person to forget some of the usual foreplay or affection that you have always engaged in. Or, after making love, the person may immediately get up and do something else, leaving you feeling alone or abandoned.

It's also possible that the person with AD will become particularly demanding sexually. He or she might have a heightened desire for sex, at the same time that you, the over-burdened caregiver, are experiencing less interest in sex.

None of these things may happen, but if they do, it could affect how you feel about continuing a sexual relationship with the affected person. If you feel that your sexual relationship is no longer satisfying and you are reluctant to continue it, you can find new ways of relating to your spouse. In the area of sexuality, as in other areas, your obligation to your partner should be balanced with your obligation to yourself.

## When You Are the Patient's Child

If your mother or father has Alzheimer's disease and your other parent is no longer alive or able to care for the affected person, you may feel you must become the primary caregiver. You probably have other important priorities in your life besides the care of your parent—such as your marriage or other significant relationship, your children, and your career. Before accepting the role as primary caregiver for your parent with Alzheimer's, examine your responsibilities carefully and see where you can cut back. The demands on your time might simply be too much.

Another consideration is whether or not your parent will live in your home. If an alternative, such as paid caregivers in a residential center for seniors or some sort of assisted-living facility are financially and emotionally possible, that may be a better solution for you. If not, understand that in caring for an AD patient in your home, you are taking on a very substantial responsibility.

If you have become the primary caregiver for your mother or father with AD and you have brothers or sisters, you should try to get as much help as you can from them. For example, if your parent lives with you and you are taking care of the day-to-day responsibilities, one sibling might be willing to take care of the bills and another the medical and dental appointments. You may not be able to share things equally, but you can still look for ways that each sibling can provide some help. As time goes on, you will be grateful for every bit of assistance that other people can provide.

It is critical for you to take care of yourself in order to avoid burnout, depression, or physical illness. The impact on a person's immune system from chronic stress—such as that often experienced by primary caregivers—has been linked to many illnesses, from the common cold to serious conditions such as heart disease. Several studies have shown that AD caregivers, as compared with noncaregivers, are at a greater risk for immune impairment. You can keep your immune system strong, however, by making sure that you take care of yourself.

Not only will caring for a parent with AD take a great deal of your time and physical stamina, it will also affect you emotionally. You may not feel comfortable making decisions for your parent and you may feel angry or guilty that you have to take charge of your parent, who once was in charge of you. In the early stage of the disease, your parent may resist your help, which might anger or otherwise upset you. It's important to deal with those feelings, not ignore them. Your feelings may be complicated by old, unresolved issues in your relationship with your parent. Later in this chapter and in Chapter 12, "How Do You Survive Stage 2?" we'll talk about ways of dealing with your feelings.

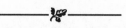

A study surveyed 252 female caregivers, 103 of whom were wives of men with Alzheimer's disease and 149 of whom were daughters caring for a parent with Alzheimer's. The study found that the daughters were significantly more likely to become clinically depressed. This may be a result of several factors. First, in marrying, a spouse commits to caring for her partner "in sickness and in health," but a daughter never signs up to care for her parents—in fact, it is the other way around. Second, a daughter may have other family responsibilities and relationships that suffer as a result of the time and stress involved in caring for her parent with AD.

You may have agreed to take care of your parent because you love him or her, because you feel it is your duty, or for other reasons. Whatever the reason, you may not have initially realized the enormity of the task you have taken on. As time goes by, even though you feel you are handling things, watch for signs of your own stress. Don't try to be a super-child. Think of taking care of yourself as an essential part of taking care of your parent with AD.

## One Caregiver's Journey

"My case is different from many others. My mother was a wonderful woman, but she wasn't a very nurturing mother. When I was younger, I didn't get along with her very well. Then I went through analysis and decided that I wanted to get along with her, and that only I could do it. She wasn't about to change, so I did. After that, we were on good terms. I never really had a close emotional bond with her, however. Many years later, when she got Alzheimer's, I took care of her and I felt a strong responsibility and obligation, but I never felt the pangs you feel when you really love somebody. If my father had gotten Alzheimer's, I would have been a basket case. I don't know how I could have stood that. I don't think I could have ever put him in a facility. I might have had him live with us even though it would have been horrible.

"When you love your parent so much, you can't bear to see him or her in that condition. You can't bear to lose your connection with him or her—which you will because, with Alzheimer's, he or she no longer has the ability to stay emotionally connected. I was fond of my mother, but I didn't have that deep bond or connection. And, fortunately, I also didn't hate her. People who hate their parents, who haven't come to terms with whatever conflict they have with a parent also have a very difficult time. They have a huge responsibility that goes on for years, and the whole time they are full of resentment. So, I think it was easier for me because of my relationship with my mother. I survived by being more detached."

# Acknowledge Your Feelings

At some point during the years of caring for a person with Alzheimer's, an estimated one half of all caregivers become clinically depressed. More than two thirds of caregivers call the job frustrating, draining, and painful. Because of their isolation, caregivers are often filled with powerful feelings that they don't have the opportunity to express. Holding in these feelings and not acknowledging them can lead to physical illness as well as depression. What are some of the ways you can acknowledge and express your feelings?

## Join a Support Group

If you haven't joined a caregiver's support group yet, join one. No one will understand what you are going through better than those who are in the same situation. Other caregivers will understand when a seemingly innocent comment by the person with AD or a family member is deeply painful to you. They can empathize with your exhaustion and can laugh with you at some of the exasperating things the person with Alzheimer's says or does.

Being in a support group will help you feel that you are not alone. Strong bonds of friendship and mutual support often develop among caregivers who participate in support groups. You will be able to discuss your feelings in the group and outside of it with the new friends you will make. You will be able to get help resolving specific problems and improving your skills as a caregiver. And you will be able to help others by sharing your ideas and experiences.

Finding the right support group for you depends on where you live. In larger cities, there are a variety of groups to choose from. There are discussion groups that give participants a chance to talk about their feelings as well as practical issues. And there are educational support groups, which are more like classes that focus on information about the disease and practical strategies needed to cope with the stress of caregiving, such as time-management techniques, communication, and

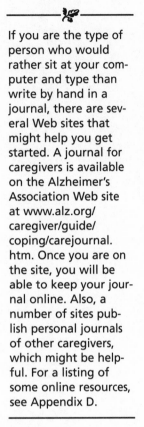

If you are the type of person who would rather sit at your computer and type than write by hand in a journal, there are several Web sites that might help you get started. A journal for caregivers is available on the Alzheimer's Association Web site at www.alz.org/ caregiver/guide/ coping/carejournal. htm. Once you are on the site, you will be able to keep your journal online. Also, a number of sites publish personal journals of other caregivers, which might be helpful. For a listing of some online resources, see Appendix D.

ways to relax. These groups are particularly valuable for those coping with the early stage of Alzheimer's disease.

In some cities, there are support groups that are designed especially for caregivers with things in common—such as members of various ethnic groups or gay or lesbian partners of AD sufferers. In less-populated areas, there may be fewer choices, but some type of support group is still very valuable. Although they do not replace the friendship and camaraderie you will experience with face-to-face communication, there are also online chat groups, which may help you express your feelings and provide you with an emotional support system. Join the type of group that is right for you, but don't hesitate to join a support group.

## Keep a Journal

It's also a good idea to keep a journal of your feelings. Write everything down, particularly your negative feelings—your anger, impatience, frustration, guilt, or any other feelings you have. Write about the situations that upset you. Putting feelings on paper provides some distance between you and your negative thoughts.

After you have written about how you feel or about a situation that upsets you, ask yourself some questions about what you are feeling and write the answers in your journal. Writing the answers will help you to examine and get some perspective on your feelings. If, for example, it's anger you are feeling about a particular incident: What are you really angry about? What could have been different in the situation? How much of what happened is a result of the disease? How much of what happened is something you could change in the future? If you can't change what happened, can you change how you are looking at the situation? Can you change how you are feeling about it? How do you feel now that you have had the chance to write about it?

## Keep Your Sense of Humor

As a caregiver for someone with one of the most awful and devastating diseases that can affect us, it might be all too easy to focus on the negative things and the unfairness of life. If you want to survive, however, you will have to train yourself to focus on the positive.

## Laughter

Humor and positive feelings have enormous physical and emotional healing power. Norman Cousins, in his book *Anatomy of an Illness*, describes his battle with a rare degenerative disease and how he laughed his way to recovery. He said that laughter is so beneficial physically that it is like "inner jogging." His theory and the result of many studies suggests that there are many positive physical benefits to be gained from laughter—it actually releases hormones in the brain, called endorphins, that act as tension-releasers, pain-reducers, breathing-improvers, and mood-elevators.

The average child laughs 400 times a day, while the average adult only laughs 15 times each day. Why have we limited our laughter so drastically, even though it feels so good and is so good for us? As adults, we have a lot more responsibilities than we did as children and, as we pile on responsibilities, we tend to take life a lot more seriously—perhaps too seriously. And who has more responsibilities than a caregiver for a person with Alzheimer's?

The good news is that there is nothing to prevent you from laughing more than 15 times a day. Although nothing is funny about the destruction the disease causes in your loved one's brain, life is still filled with humorous moments if you are willing to recognize them. The key is to not miss those moments. Even though your family has to deal with a tragic disease, it's still okay to laugh and have good times.

Start by noticing how often you laugh each day and try to increase the number of moments of laughter as much as you can. One way to increase your daily dose of laughter is to write on a card, which you place in a conspicuous place: How many times have we laughed today? Laughter is even better when it is shared, so laugh with the person with AD. Even though later in the disease he or she may not completely understand the joke or funny situation, it will lift his or her spirits to see you laugh.

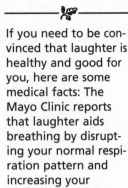

If you need to be convinced that laughter is healthy and good for you, here are some medical facts: The Mayo Clinic reports that laughter aids breathing by disrupting your normal respiration pattern and increasing your breathing rate. It can even help clear mucus from your lungs. Laughter is also good for your heart. It increases circulation and improves the delivery of oxygen and nutrients to tissues throughout your body. A good laugh helps your immune system fight off colds, flu, and sinus problems by increasing the concentration of cells that function as antibodies in your saliva. And it may help control pain by raising the levels of certain brain chemicals (endorphins). It is also a natural stress reliever. Have you ever laughed so hard that you doubled over, almost fell off your chair, or had to spit out your food? That's because you can't maintain muscle tension when you are laughing.

Also, try to see the humor in being a caregiver. Be willing to laugh at yourself and your situation. Share the ridiculous moments that happen with your friends in your Alzheimer's support group. If you tell a funny story, you get to laugh again, the person hearing it gets to laugh, and you feel even better because you've helped someone else.

When you schedule a moment to relax, read funny books, magazines, or joke books. Listen to tapes, see movies, television shows, or videos that make you laugh. Go to funny Web sites, visit a comedy club, or tune into Comedy Central. Call up people who lift your spirits and have good senses of humor.

As you continue to consciously find ways to increase your laughter—or inner jogging—you will begin to notice your stress level decreasing. You are bound to feel better, you will cope with problems more effectively, and people will enjoy being around you.

## Fun

What about fun? We all have different activities that we consider fun. Don't let yourself get so overwhelmed with the care of the person with AD that you forget to have fun. Make a list of things that are fun for you. Is playing tennis or another sport on the list? How about playing cards or other games with friends? Going to a movie? Going on an outing to a park, a beach, or a lake? Don't neglect the fun activities in your life just because you have become a caregiver.

Continue to pursue activities and social contacts outside your home. It may not be easy to schedule these activities, but the rewards for having balance in your life are worth it. Meeting your own needs by taking time to have some fun will satisfy you and give you additional strength for your caregiving tasks.

No matter how great our responsibilities, we all deserve to have fun. Even if you never took time for fun before, to survive the long and difficult challenges ahead in caring for someone with Alzheimer's, make yourself take time to have fun now.

# Ask for Help!

Caregivers are often "take-charge" people who feel that they can handle things on their own. They feel comfortable taking care of people, but don't feel comfortable asking other people to help them. Taking care of someone with Alzheimer's disease, however, is not something anyone can do successfully without help. It is just too much. If you are a take-charge type of person, try to recognize that this situation is different from other ones in your life, and you will need to ask for help.

Other caregivers don't ask for help because they are afraid that those they ask might turn down their request. Of course, it hurts to be rejected, but don't let a fear of rejection stop you from asking for help. People may refuse your request for help for a number of reasons. Some simply may not want to help. Others may want to help, but have very legitimate reasons for saying no. The person you ask may, in fact, feel quite bad about having to say no. Whatever the reason for the rejection, don't let it stop you from asking someone else for help. Many people may be willing to help, but they need to be asked first.

You might be more successful in getting help if you ask for something specific rather than tossing out a general question like, "Do you think you could help me sometime?" Ask for something you think the person is capable of giving, given who they are. For example, if your neighbor likes to shop, perhaps she wouldn't mind picking up a few groceries for you each week.

## Getting Time Off

About two thirds of caregivers are reluctant to leave their loved one alone even for brief periods of time. The first step in getting time off is recognizing how important it is for you to do so. If you feel guilty about taking time away from the person with Alzheimer's, you won't get the help you need. You are, in fact, doing the person a favor by taking time off for yourself. When you return and are emotionally and physically refreshed, you will not only feel better, but, because a person

—————❦—————

The help of family or friends can sometimes be a mixed blessing. Although visits may give you time off or provide help with chores, the helper may criticize the way you provide care. Remember that the person is only responding to what he or she sees at that moment, not the whole situation. His or her criticism may also come from guilt about not helping more. Try not to react in anger. Listen to suggestions, but simply disregard what isn't possible or necessary to change.

with Alzheimer's is typically very sensitive to a caregiver's mood, he or she will also feel better.

In order to get the time off, however, you will have to ask for help. Again, don't make a general request, but ask a relative or friend to spend a particular number of hours a week or a month with the person with AD so you can take a break.

## Getting Professional Help

You may have to ask for help not only with certain tasks or to get time off, but also to understand and deal with the emotions you are feeling. Depression and other negative feelings can be a real problem for caregivers. Sixty percent of caregivers show clinical symptoms of depression. You may be suffering from depression without even being aware if it. There are a number of signs of depression to watch for. They include the following:

- Feelings of hopelessness
- Feelings of guilt or worthlessness
- Feelings of sadness
- Loss of interest in activities you once enjoyed
- Suicidal thoughts
- Difficulty concentrating, thinking, or making decisions
- Weight loss or weight gain
- Chronic headaches or other chronic pains
- Insomnia

If you experience several of the above symptoms within a number of weeks, there is a good chance that you may be clinically depressed. If so, it is important that you seek the help of a professional. Even if you thought you could handle the stress of caregiving, the actual day-to-day experience may be a very difficult emotional adjustment. Seeing a therapist, even for only a few weeks, can often provide relief. A therapist can help you understand and resolve the grief and other emotions you are feeling, which will then cause your depression to lift.

If nondrug approaches such as therapy don't help, you could ask your doctor about antidepressant medications. The person with AD may already be taking one of these drugs. Antidepressants usually do help relieve depression, but they often have a number of side effects. Also, drugs are not a substitute for taking care of yourself in other ways.

## Exercise and Eat Well

As a caregiver, you need to keep fit now more than ever. You have to function for two people, not just one, and you have to stay in shape to do it. Part of staying is shape is eating right. Good food is the fuel your body needs to keep caregiving. Skipping meals, eating poorly, or drinking lots of caffeine will not work. Learn to prepare and eat simple, nutritious, well-balanced meals. Stay away from lots of sugar and avoid having more than two to three ounces of alcohol daily.

Exercise is the other part of staying in shape. It has beneficial effects on just about everything, including your mood, your stamina, and your memory. Like laughter, exercise can release endorphins that will lift your mood. Exercise will help you sleep and keep your immune system strong so you can fight off colds and other illnesses. As we said in an earlier chapter, exercise is also something that is important for the person with AD to do regularly, so it's wise to plan times to exercise together.

The most common reason people don't exercise is that they feel they don't have enough time to do so. Finding time to exercise can certainly be a problem, but the good news is that short-duration exercise that adds up to 30 minutes a day can work as well as longer, more strenuous workouts. You don't need to drive to the gym and get on the machines for 40 minutes to exercise. A few minutes of walking, then some gardening or dancing to your favorite tune, mixed with running up and down the stairs will work if it all adds up to at least 30 minutes a day.

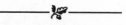

What if you feel you are too old or too inactive to start exercising? Or what if you have a medical problem that limits you? First, you are never too old to begin doing some exercise. Many seniors who never exercised when they were younger have started exercise programs that are extremely beneficial. If you have some medical problem or chronic condition, exercise may actually help your condition, but consult your doctor about what exercise regimen is right for you.

Keep in shape and keep your spirits up, because with Alzheimer's disease, the challenges of a caregiver only get harder. One caregiver commented that the key to coping successfully with the responsibilities of caring for a person with AD is to realize that it is impossible. If you recognize that the task is impossible to do perfectly, then you can just try to do the best you can.

# 10

# What to Expect in Stage 2

―――――――――― ❧ ――――――――――

As Chapter 7, "What to Expect in Stage 1," discussed, the division of Alzheimer's disease into stages is somewhat arbitrary and there is overlap among the different stages. During Stage 1—which usually lasts between one and four years— many people are diagnosed with the disease, particularly as awareness of AD spreads and more families understand the benefits of an early diagnosis. Many affected people, however, may not be diagnosed with Alzheimer's disease until they are already in Stage 2.

The second or middle stage is generally the longest stage of AD. It usually lasts between 2 and 10 years, and sometimes as long as 12 years. The brain damage that began in the early stages of AD has progressed significantly by Stage 2, limiting the affected person's abilities even more. By the time the person with Alzheimer's reaches the second stage, the signs, symptoms, and behaviors that are common in the early stages are magnified many times.

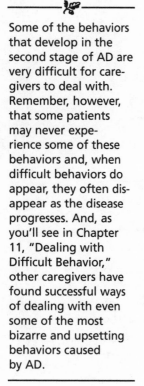

Some of the behaviors that develop in the second stage of AD are very difficult for caregivers to deal with. Remember, however, that some patients may never experience some of these behaviors and, when difficult behaviors do appear, they often disappear as the disease progresses. And, as you'll see in Chapter 11, "Dealing with Difficult Behavior," other caregivers have found successful ways of dealing with even some of the most bizarre and upsetting behaviors caused by AD.

# Some General Changes

In the early stage of Alzheimer's, the affected person might seem fine one moment and then display behaviors of the disease the next. In the second stage, however, you will rarely see completely normal functioning anymore. Instead, throughout the course of the day, the affected person may move from behaviors more characteristic of the early stage to behaviors more typical of the middle stage.

During the second stage of AD, an affected person will usually lose the awareness of her condition that she may have once had. Despite daily evidence of profound memory loss, she will generally deny that she has any memory problems. If you point out an example of her forgetfulness, she will usually make an excuse. She might say that she was so busy she just forgot or that she simply can't be bothered with every detail. She is unaware of her errors most of the time. The good news is that she is no longer very worried about her condition or concerned that you and other relatives are upset over it.

In Stage 2, as in Stage 1, rummaging and saving useless items are common behaviors. Some people will also begin to have auditory and visual hallucinations. Most will exhibit various types of repetitive verbal or physical behaviors and have much shorter attention spans. Judgment and decision-making, which require organizing thoughts and thinking logically, are abilities that are also greatly diminished in this stage. Most people in this stage will no longer be able to handle money at all, even to make simple purchases.

With increased difficulties in many areas, the person with AD will become more and more dependent on you, the caregiver, and more isolated socially. Certain behaviors and personality traits may not be affected, but most patients will still need full-time supervision at this stage.

## One Caregiver's Journey

"When my mother was still at the senior residential home, the manager called and said that she had not been down for meals for two days. I was upset that he hadn't called right away, but he said they thought she was with me. When I got there, she wasn't in the apartment, and no one could find her. I had visions of her on the street somewhere, so I went to the police, who said that the first thing they do is search the entire premises. They came back to the residential hotel and started on the top floor of 14 floors. They finally found her in the stairwell on the third floor. She was just sitting there. She had been sitting on the stairs for two days! I was very upset, but she wasn't. She just said 'hello' to me as if everything was normal.

"Although she seemed confused, she wasn't at all frightened. I still don't know what happened. She hadn't fallen. She wasn't hurt. Maybe she had a small stroke, forgot what she was doing, and just sat down. My mother was always very physically active and would never take an elevator if she could take the stairs. By now, she had a Safe Return bracelet, but it didn't matter in this instance. Nobody else in the building walked the stairs, so nobody found her. Afterwards, I cleaned her up and took her to the emergency room. They did some tests but couldn't see evidence of a stroke or anything else. It was probably just Alzheimer's disease."

An Alzheimer's patient may stand in front of a mirror, talking to herself. When this happens, it's likely that she is unable to recognize herself in the mirror. She may carry on a conversation, completely unaware that she is talking to herself. This is often called the "mirror sign"—a sign of the progression of the disease. Since she's unable to recognize herself, it's perhaps easier for you to understand why she also has trouble recognizing family, neighbors, or friends.

## Severe Memory Loss

In the second stage of the disease, memory loss becomes much more severe, and defects in memory, retention, and recall become more obvious even to a casual observer. Right after finishing lunch, for example, the person with AD may ask, "Did we have lunch yet?" During this stage, memory loss also begins to affect long-term memory as well as short-term memory.

The increased memory loss and confusion in the person with AD in turn affects many areas of life. The affected person will have more and more problems retaining new information, recalling familiar people or events, doing any sort of calculations, making decisions, planning, or following stories and plots in conversations, television shows, or books.

Although the affected person may be able to talk about familiar topics such as the weather, she may be unaware of losing her train of thought in the middle of a conversation. She may forget to initiate or complete normal routines, including daily hygiene routines (see later in this chapter). She might forget to take medication or to turn off the stove or running water.

Other common results of increased memory loss in Stage 2 include the following signs, some of which may have already begun in Stage 1:

- Forgets appointments and socially significant events
- Is unaware of what happened yesterday
- Is unable to plan tomorrow
- Asks the same question repeatedly
- Can't remember visits immediately after you leave
- Has problems recognizing close friends and/or family
- Is disoriented about time—confuses day and night or merges past with present
- Forgets learned social behaviors, such as manners
- Is disoriented even in familiar surroundings
- Has problems with reading, numbers, following written signs, writing his name, adding, or subtracting

### One Caregiver's Journey

"One thing was upsetting to me even though, by now, I was really used to everything changing. I went to visit my mother on my birthday and said to her, 'Mother, do you know what day this is?' She said 'What?' I said 'It's August fifth!' assuming she would remember the day she gave birth to me. She said, 'Oh, is it summer already?' For me, it was kind of a shock that she didn't remember my birthday."

# Difficulty Communicating

The severe memory loss in this stage, in turn, makes it more difficult for the person with AD to communicate with other people. Communication is a two-way process—sending and receiving information. People with Alzheimer's have trouble both speaking and understanding when spoken to. The problems in both areas become much more pronounced in Stage 2.

## Difficulty Speaking

As you learned in Chapter 2, "When to Worry: The Ten Warning Signs of Alzheimer's," people in the early stage of AD begin to have difficulty finding the correct word for an object. The medical term for this is anomia—when the affected person still knows that a book is a book, for example, but has trouble accessing the word "book."

By the second stage of the disease, an AD patient begins to have substantial anomia, especially relating to abstract, more specific, or less familiar words. To compensate for not being able to find the right words, the person may use related words—words that are similar, but not the right words. He or she may also begin to "fill in" with sounds or gibberish instead of words. The conversation of the affected person may thus become progressively more vague and confusing to you. The person might also make up stories that he or she tells over and over again as a kind of compensation for not being able to converse coherently.

The affected person will also develop more noticeable agnosia by the second stage of the disease, which is characterized by not only forgetting the word for a familiar object, but also not recognizing the object at all. For example, the person looks at a book and doesn't know what it is anymore. Agnosia may be present to a limited degree in the early stage of AD, but you may not notice it because at first it only affects relatively unfamiliar things. In the middle stage of the disease, however, agnosia becomes much more pronounced. Although the affected person may continue to use relatively good grammar and diction, the inability to recognize familiar things affects

As language skills diminish, an AD patient may often use body language and nonverbal behavior to express herself. Because she isn't speaking much, it's important that you don't then begin to talk about her in her presence as though she isn't there. Just because she is having difficulty speaking doesn't mean she can't still understand what is being said. Remember to respect the patient and not treat her as an object, regardless of the level of her language abilities.

his or her capacity to have a simple conversation and also interferes with other daily activities.

One of the most disturbing aspects of agnosia is the inability to recognize people. Your loved one with AD may not recognize you. He or she may accuse you of being an intruder or may think you are someone else. This problem will usually start with people the affected person hasn't seen in a while and then progress to even those closest to him or her.

Some of the other communication problems that you may notice in Stage 2 in the person with AD:

- Seems unable to concentrate
- Hesitates when responding verbally
- Speaks more slowly
- Loses his or her train of thought frequently
- Rarely initiates a conversation
- Withdraws from most social situations
- Asks fewer questions
- Endlessly repeats ideas, questions, or words
- Cannot tell you what he or she needs

## Difficulty Understanding Speech

By Stage 2, people with Alzheimer's have problems understanding what even those closest to them are saying. Caregivers and family members often misinterpret this lack of understanding and believe that the person is being stubborn or uncooperative. You may say you are going out and will be right back. Your loved one with AD appears to understand and may even say, "Okay" or "I understand." But, in fact, the person doesn't understand. He or she might get very upset and start looking for you as soon as you leave.

In the second stage of AD, some forms of communication also become more difficult for the person with AD to understand. A person who would understand something being said to him face to face may not understand the same conversation on the telephone. A person with AD may understand his caregiver, who speaks slowly and maintains direct eye contact, but might not understand a fast-talking relative. He may also be easily distracted by noise or multiple speakers.

Some examples of the problems with understanding in the second stage of AD include:

- The inability to follow a simple request
- Trouble understanding ordinary conversation
- Difficulty focusing and maintaining attention
- The need for repetition of simple directions
- The inability to understand the meaning of what is read
- The inability to understand facial cues

Your doctor may term the difficulties that the person with AD is having with communication aphasia, which is when the brain deteriorates enough to impair the speech process. There are two types of aphasias—expressive aphasia, when the patient can't express himself even though he understands what is said and receptive aphasia, when the patient is unable to understand what he hears. With other types of dementia, such as multi-infarct disease, often only one part of the brain is affected, allowing the person, for example, to understand but not be able to express himself. With AD, however, it is more likely that the aphasia will eventually affect both speech and comprehension.

## Physical Changes

Since Alzheimer's disease can affect many parts of the brain, people with AD may begin to lose some physical coordination as the disease progresses. They may start to have perceptual motor problems and problems carrying out purposeful movements. For example, the affected person may have difficulty getting into a chair, setting the dinner table, or managing buttons and zippers.

Apraxia is the medical name for the inability to carry out purposeful movements and actions. It occurs when the brain

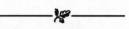

Before you assume that the person with AD cannot understand what you have to say, make sure that he or she can hear you. Many older people have hearing loss that can interfere with conversational ability. Get the person's hearing tested. Also, ask the doctor to check the wax in the person's ears. Removing earwax often results in a remarkable improvement. If the person wears a hearing aid, check the batteries regularly to make sure they are working.

———— ✿ ————

An early warning sign that a person with AD is developing the loss of coordination from apraxia is a change in her handwriting. Later, she may become slightly unsteady when walking. As the damage from AD causes further apraxia, she may walk with a slow, shuffling gait. When these physical coordination problems develop, be sure to provide handrails and other types of support for the unsteady person and be patient with her ability to do anything that requires good coordination.

signal to a part of the body is not able to get through to the muscles in that area. So, even though the muscles are still functional, the connection between the brain and the muscles is not working.

In the first stage of AD, apraxia may have been present, but it may have only affected more complex tasks. As the disease progresses into the second and third stages, the patient may develop increased apraxia, which will leave him unable to perform simple tasks, such as feeding or washing himself, even though he has no muscle weakness. In Stage 1, a person with AD might have difficulty when faced with a lot of choices of what to wear, but if the clothes were laid out, he or she was able to get dressed alone. In Stage 2, however, the affected person may no longer have the coordination to be able to get dressed without help.

In Stage 2, patients with Alzheimer's disease also become more and more restless. They dislike being in one place and seem to need to keep moving. The affected person might pace around the room or outside, as though searching for something. The wandering behavior that might have developed in Stage 1 becomes more pronounced in Stage 2. In this stage, the affected person may wander for hours before becoming tired.

An AD patient's restlessness may be worse in the late afternoon and at night. Many Alzheimer's patients experience increased confusion at the end of the day when the sun goes down—a condition called sundowning. The affected person may also be more agitated, irritable, or even violent at that time of day.

Also, the person with AD may develop difficulty sleeping at night. He or she may awaken frequently at night and, each time, get up and wander. Or, the affected person may sleep more often than usual.

Not everyone experiences all of these symptoms, but some of the physical changes that are common in Stage 2 of Alzheimer's disease include:

- Poor spatial orientation
- Poor coordination
- Poor dexterity
- A wide gait
- A tendency to trip
- Slight difficulty chewing and swallowing
- Gaining and then losing weight
- Occasional muscle twitches or jerking
- Repetitive movements
- Aimless wandering and restlessness, especially at night

## Personality Changes

In Stage 2, the patient's personality, which in Stage 1 was changing somewhat, may become increasingly apathetic. The affected person may become more self-absorbed and show little concern for family or friends. He or she will be likely to withdraw socially more and more.

In addition to the tendency to withdraw, a disturbing personality change in many Alzheimer patients is increasing paranoia and suspicion. This may begin in Stage 1 or in Stage 2, or it may not occur at all in some people. A common example is when a person with AD loses something and then accuses his caregiver of stealing the item. Or, an affected person may refuse to eat a meal because he thinks you are trying to poison him. If the person is your spouse, he may accuse you of having an affair.

Other changes in personality that you might observe in Stage 2 include when the Alzheimer's patient:

- Is easily agitated
- Has wide mood swings
- Is extremely anxious
- Cries easily
- Acts childish or silly
- Is irritable or fidgety

Sleep patterns change with aging so that older persons not only sleep fewer hours, but also usually spend less time in deep, restful sleep and in REM or dream sleep. In addition to these age-associated changes in sleep patterns, people with AD experience abnormal disruptions in their sleep patterns. AD patients spend a very high percentage of their time in light sleep and less time in deep sleep. They often awaken frequently in the night. Some may experience circadian rhythm disturbances—like people with jet lag—which may keep them awake at night and asleep during the day. Sundowning may also be related to circadian rhythm disorders.

- Has hallucinations or delusions
- Talks to imaginary people
- Engages in inappropriate social behaviors
- Resents interference by caregivers
- Has angry catastrophic reactions

*One Caregiver's Journey*

"My mother never really got paranoid, but I know that a lot of people with Alzheimer's do. A friend of mine, whose husband has AD, took him to a convenience store with her one day. He went right up to the clerk and told her that my friend was trying to kidnap him. My friend explained to the clerk that he was her husband, and he had Alzheimer's disease. The clerk handled it very well. She calmly listened to my friend's husband and told him not to worry, she would watch out for him. Then she distracted him by getting him interested in some product on the shelf. Soon he was calm again and had forgotten that he was in danger of being kidnapped by his wife."

## The Hygiene Nightmare

One of the most upsetting problems for caregivers is when the person with AD begins to neglect his or her health and personal hygiene habits. Chapters 18, "Mealtime Traumas," and 19, "Personal Hygiene at Home," present many good ideas for dealing with problems in these two areas. Following, however, are some of the hygiene and mealtime problems that are likely to develop in Stage 2.

Because we learned personal hygiene habits as children and have been doing them all of our lives, we don't realize the necessary mental functioning needed to carry out many seemingly simple tasks, such as dressing, using the toilet, bathing, and even eating. As the brain damage from AD continues, affected people become less able to initiate purposeful activity and to sequence events, both of which are required for eating and taking care of one's personal hygiene.

# Eating

Eating is essential to life and health, and it is also a very social activity. Just as AD affects other social activities, the person with AD becomes unable to participate in meals in the same socially acceptable way. Memory impairment and loss of impulse control and coordination from the disease makes the eating process difficult for people with AD. In Stage 2, for example, the person with AD may forget when his last meal was eaten. He may develop a huge appetite for junk food. He or she may refuse food offered to him or her, but then insist on eating other people's food. Or the person may gradually lose all interest in food.

In regard to the actual process of eating, in Stage 2 the person with AD may begin to use table utensils improperly, forget table manners entirely, or develop sloppier ones. Also, at this stage, some people may develop difficulty chewing and swallowing. See Chapter 18 for more information on how to deal with eating difficulties.

# Personal Hygiene

By Stage 2, most AD patients have difficulty dressing. Many have begun to wear the wrong clothes or to wear several layers of clothing. Some patients may undress at inappropriate times or in the wrong place. As we discussed earlier, some of the difficulty dressing is a result of the loss of coordination caused by the disease.

Many patients also begin to have difficulty bathing and grooming. Some develop a fear of showering or bathing and put up a lot of resistance to bathing. Others are willing to bathe, but only with assistance. Patients will also neglect brushing their teeth and flossing. If the person with AD has dentures, he or she will no longer be able to take care of them without assistance.

Finally, some patients develop incontinence in this stage, although others may not develop this problem until Stage 3. Some people will only have occasional accidents in the second

Upset when your loved one with AD won't shower? Be patient with her. She probably has several reasons for resisting bathing. She might have trouble finding the bathroom. She might find the water temperature too hot or too cold or fear slipping or falling in the water. She might have forgotten why she needs to bathe. With her loss of coordination, she might find the task too difficult and be embarrassed about accepting help. Or, she might be depressed.

stage of Alzheimer's, but others may become completely in-continent. Incontinence can occur because the person with AD forgets where the bathroom is or forgets that he or she has to use the toilet. Or the person may no longer connect the sensation of having to go to the bathroom with the knowledge of what to do about it. There may be a medical cause for incontinence that can be treated, so this condition should be discussed with the affected person's doctor as soon as it occurs.

# 11

# *Dealing with Difficult Behavior*

―――――――――― ❧ ――――――――――

Why do Alzheimer's patients develop behaviors that are so difficult for caregivers to handle? Why do they repeat questions over and over, follow you around, act suspicious of you, or have catastrophic emotional reactions? To understand why AD patients do these things, remember that the world the person lives in is more and more limited as the disease progresses. The Alzheimer's patient can do fewer and fewer tasks. Why shouldn't he or she repeat them? The affected person recognizes fewer faces and places, and remembers less and less. Why shouldn't his or her fears increase?

As we discussed in Chapter 8, "General Guidelines for Caring for Alzheimer's Patients," it will help you care for a person with AD if you can have respect and compassion for him or her. When dealing with difficult behaviors, it's especially important to be compassionate and remember that such behaviors are not intentional and designed to annoy you, but are the result of the disease. In addition to being compassionate, there are, of course, many practical things you can do when your loved one displays behaviors that upset you. You don't have to just let his or her actions disrupt your life. In this chapter, you'll learn how to deal with difficult behaviors, based on creative ways other caregivers have handled them.

———————— 🦋 ————————

Be careful about what you talk about around a person with Alzheimer's. You may inadvertently contribute to repetitive questioning on the part of the person with AD by discussing plans for various activities or appointments in advance of the actual event. It is best not to mention an outing or activity until just prior to getting ready to leave for the event. That will keep the person from asking about it days ahead of time.

---

*One Caregiver's Journey*

"A woman in my support group told us about her husband with AD. He would get catalogs and send away for everything in them. He was sending for stuff almost every day, and she had to make regular trips to the post office to return things. She tried to get to the mail ahead of him to hide the catalogs, but couldn't always do it. The group had a number of suggestions, such as changing their address to the neighbor's address or getting a post office box. She didn't want to do either. Finally, when she couldn't stand it anymore, she got a post office box. That's usually what people do. They suffer through these things until they can't take it anymore—but they don't have to."

## Repetition

There are two kinds of repetitive behaviors that develop in Alzheimer's patients—repeating words, phrases, or questions and repeating certain behaviors. A person with AD may develop both problems, or neither.

### Already Asked and Answered

Repetitive questions may be a result of forgetting that the question was already asked and answered, or it may be an indication that the person with AD has a problem or needs reassurance of some sort. As an affected person's ability to communicate diminishes, she may not be able to say exactly what she means. You may have to try to figure out what she is really asking. For example, if she continually asks, "What's for dinner?" perhaps she is hungry and you can offer her a snack. Or perhaps she was always the one who planned dinner and now you have taken over that responsibility. She may feel uncertain that you are really doing the job. You could ease her anxiety by writing out the menu for each night's dinner so she could see that you have, in fact, planned dinner.

In other cases, the affected person may feel threatened by your answer to her question, so she might repeat it, hoping for a different answer. She might, for example, repeatedly ask when she is going to the doctor because going to the doctor is frightening for her.

If you think that the repeated question or phrase itself isn't particularly meaningful, perhaps the person is trying to express a concern but can't find the right words. He or she may not be able to tell you about a physical problem or a particular worry, and the resulting anxiety may come out in repetitious questions or phrases. If you can figure out what the problem is, then you may be able fix it or at least address it directly.

If you can't discover any particular fear or anxiety, perhaps the affected person just needs some extra reassurance. When trying to reassure the person, always use a calm voice, direct eye contact, and brief, simple statements, and make sure to respond to the emotional content of the statements, not just the words. It also might help to give the person with AD a reassuring hug or a gentle touch to let him or her know that, as far as you are concerned, everything is all right.

It's possible that the repetitious questions or words are simply a way to get your attention. In that case, it's best to just ignore the person with AD. Sometimes, not responding will make the person angry or agitated, but other times the questions will stop if the behavior doesn't get your attention. Ignoring the questions may be an especially good idea when you are annoyed—it will keep the person from hearing the anger in your tone of voice. It's still best to try to discover the meaning in the questions or words first, however, before ignoring the person.

## Been There, Done That

What about repetitious actions? There are two types of repetitious actions—those that cause problems for you and those that don't. If the person with AD wants to fold the laundry over and over, why not let him? He may feel that he is helping you with the housework. Letting him continue may make him feel he is still able to make a contribution.

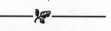

People with AD live in a confusing, overwhelming world. It is often too noisy, too cluttered, or too busy. It's filled with people the affected person may not recognize and people who do things without giving him or her time to understand what is going on. Reassuring the person that everything is all right with soothing words, a tender touch, a pat on the back, or a hug will help ease anxiety and minimize difficult behaviors.

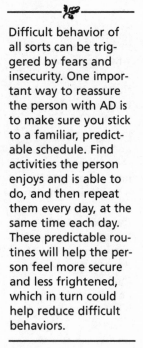

Difficult behavior of all sorts can be triggered by fears and insecurity. One important way to reassure the person with AD is to make sure you stick to a familiar, predictable schedule. Find activities the person enjoys and is able to do, and then repeat them every day, at the same time each day. These predictable routines will help the person feel more secure and less frightened, which in turn could help reduce difficult behaviors.

What if the person's "stuck in the rut" symptom is something that he or she shouldn't be doing, such as watering a plant over and over again? Not only does the behavior drive you crazy, it will kill the plant. You can't ignore it. What can you do? Try to redirect or distract the person by getting her to do something else.

## Clinging

It can be really annoying when your loved one with AD constantly follows you around. She won't entertain herself, and she seems to believe that you will leave her if she doesn't watch you constantly. Like a frightened puppy, she won't let you out of her sight. You may not even be able to go to the bathroom or take a shower without being followed.

This problem is a result of fear and insecurity triggered by the affected person's memory loss. You may represent the only security left in a confusing world, and the person with AD might only feel secure when he or she has you in clear view. The clinging behavior might also give him or her a sense of belonging and ease feelings of isolation.

What can you do about this clinging behavior? As with harmful repetitious behaviors, try to reassure the affected person with kind words, a hug, or a gentle touch. At the same time, try to distract the affected person. Get him involved in a project that he likes to do—folding clothes, listening to music, looking at a picture book, playing with a pet or whatever kind of activity will interest him for a while. That may give you time to take a shower in private—and you certainly have the right to some privacy. If you can't set him or her up with an enjoyable activity, then simply lock the bathroom door.

When you don't need privacy, it's best to just ignore the clinging behavior if you can. Many caregivers learn to accept that their loved ones will shadow every move all day long. If you remember that the person is not trying to annoy you, but is just doing the best he or she can in response to the disease, it might not get to you so much. Also, make sure that you plan time away from caregiving. If you have regular time off, you might be more tolerant of the Alzheimer's patient's clinging behavior.

## One Caregiver's Journey

"A man who had Alzheimer's, named Leonard, moved into the senior residence where my mother lived. He wasn't quite as bad as my mother was, but he took an immediate liking to her. He was just crazy about my mother and was with her all the time. My mother liked men and didn't object much. Often, Leonard even slept in her apartment. Late one night I got a phone call from her. She whispered into the phone, 'There's a strange man sleeping in my bed.' I said, 'But that's Leonard. He often stays overnight.' She said, 'I don't want him here.' I said, 'Why don't you just let him sleep there. You have two beds.' She said, 'No, I want him to go home.' I said, 'Okay, I'll come over.' When I got there, she said, 'Talk quietly, you'll wake him.' I said, 'Well, if you want me to send him home, I have to wake him. Are you sure you want him to go?' She said 'Yes.' So I went into the bedroom and woke him up. He was a little cross, but he got up and went to his apartment."

## Suspiciousness and Paranoia

Your loved one with Alzheimer's might suddenly accuse you of all sorts of evil behavior. He or she may proclaim, "You're stealing from me." Or, "You're out to get me." Unreasonable suspicions and accusations can be very hurtful to you, particularly since you are devoting so much of your life to the person's care.

Suspicion and resulting accusations, however, are simply a response to the affected person's diminishing control of the world around her. She is less sure of what is happening. Her interpretations of what she sees and hears and her reasoning abilities are less reliable. She misplaces things, and when they are missing assumes that you have stolen them. It's the disease that leads the affected person to interpret events from a paranoid or threatening point of view and then to lash out, usually at those he or she is closest to—and, as the caregiver, that's you.

Dealing with insults and accusations can be even more difficult when you are out in public with the affected person. Some caregivers find it helpful to wear signs that say: "My father has Alzheimer's, please direct your questions to me." If you don't want to wear a sign, just tell the person your loved one is talking to that he or she has Alzheimer's and that insults and suspicion are part of the disease. Also, be sure to explain to other family members and people who work for you that suspicious accusations are a part of the disease and not to be taken personally.

As with repetitive questions, there might be an underlying meaning to the affected person's accusations. "You're stealing from me," might really mean, "I can't find anything anymore. Why don't you help me?" If you think that's the case, rather than arguing with the person, help him or her find the missing object. Try to learn where the person's favorite hiding places are for objects that are frequently "stolen." If the person with AD suspects that money is "missing," let him or her keep small amounts of money on hand in a pocket or purse.

Once again, reassurance might work. Rather than arguing or lashing out at the AD patient who insults you, it might help to reassure him or her. Instead of saying "No one's trying to poison you," say "I know you feel frightened." Respond to the feeling behind the accusation, rather than defending yourself. Soothing and calming words or a gentle hug work better than anger and indignation.

It may also work—as with repetitious questions or behaviors—to gently change the subject, or redirect the person's attention elsewhere. This option may not be successful, however, because the person is often angry when making an accusation. Finally, you might want to talk with the person's doctor about the paranoid behaviors. Adjustments may be needed in his or her prescription medications.

## Rage and Catastrophic Outbursts

What can you do when the person with AD is verbally abusive? What if she has frequent bouts of angry, agitated behavior? In general, don't return the anger and don't argue. Try to be gentle, soothing, and reassuring. During an angry fit or catastrophic reaction, don't try to restrain the person, but keep dangerous objects out of reach.

Again, try to look for the reason the angry outburst has occurred and for patterns. Is there too much noise or activity? You may need to reduce the clutter, the noise, or the number of people in the house. Has there been a shift in the ordinary schedule or routine so that the person has had to handle unexpected and stressful events? Make sure there hasn't been some upsetting change in the room—like missing objects or moved furniture. Does the person always get angry at night or when it's time for a bath? If you can figure out what triggers the angry behavior, you might be able to make a change that would prevent it in the future.

In addition to keeping noise, clutter, and changes at a minimum, how can you avoid angry outbursts? If he is more agitated at night, for example, you might get a night-light to help reduce confusion. Perhaps you can give the person more privacy while bathing or more independence in other activities. Perhaps he just needs you to listen more carefully or to acknowledge his anger and frustration over the loss of control the disease brings.

To get the angry episode to end, try distracting the affected person with some activity she enjoys. If distraction doesn't work, try to ignore the angry behavior. If necessary, leave the room and give the person time to calm down. After it's all over, let her forget about the incident—bringing it up again will only increase anxiety.

It's a good idea to speak with the affected person's doctor about frequent angry outbursts. There may be a medical reason, or the person's medications might be causing adverse side effects. Reducing caffeine intake may also be helpful. In severe cases, the doctor will probably prescribe medication to keep the patient calm.

What if the person's behavior is physically threatening or abusive? Your first responsibility is to protect yourself and anyone else who might be in danger. If you are frightened, leave the area and stay clear of the person until the episode passes. Take with you anything that could be used as a weapon. If you feel you can't control the person, call for assistance.

## Hallucinations or Delusions

The progressive brain damage caused by AD affects an individual's ability to interpret information accurately, which can lead to hallucinations or delusions. Hallucinations are when a person actually senses something that isn't there. Delusions are false beliefs that are firmly held despite strong evidence to the contrary. About 10 to 15 percent of people with AD have hallucinations or delusions.

An affected person might seem to be talking with someone who is not present and actually see or hear the person— a hallucination—or might firmly believe a deceased person is alive—a delusion. Or, a person with AD may say someone is trying to break into the house, when all he or she has heard is a tree branch brushing against the house.

When delusions or hallucinations occur, don't argue with the person. Don't try, for example, to convince the person that his deceased spouse is not there. At the same time, don't play along with a delusion or hallucination as though it were true. You can calmly listen to the person and try to comfort him without agreeing that there is a burglar in the house.

As with other difficult behaviors, it often works to distract the person so that he forgets about the hallucination. It also works to be reassuring, both verbally and physically. Tell him that even though you don't hear the voices, you understand how frightened he must feel. Give him a hug and plenty of verbal reassurance until the episode passes.

## Depression

Mild depression is likely to occur in one third to one half of all people with Alzheimer's, and more serious depression occurs in about 10 percent of patients. In many cases, depression sets in as the person becomes more aware of his or her memory loss. In the early stages of the disease, sadness may be a result of the grieving process the person is going through after the diagnosis or as he or she becomes more aware of the disease. If this sadness is accompanied by other symptoms, the person may be depressed. In addition to feelings of sadness or despondency, other symptoms of depression include the following:

- Loss of energy or fatigue
- Apathy or listlessness
- Changes in appetite
- Loss of interest in pleasurable activities

- Sleep disturbances
- Suicidal tendencies
- Preoccupation with health, or hypochondria

It's often hard for a caregiver to tell whether the person is depressed or whether he or she is simply more apathetic or docile because of the disease. Even symptoms such as loss of appetite or sleep disturbances may be caused by Alzheimer's disease, rather than depression. Serious depression usually is characterized by a sudden deterioration in sleep, appetite, energy, and interest in daily activities, as well as threats of suicide.

If you suspect that the affected person is depressed, psychotherapy or counseling—either individual or group—might be very effective. In addition, exercise, good nutrition, and herbal medicine, such as St. John's Wort, may also help. Another natural remedy, S-adenosylmethionine (SAM-e) is considered by many to be an effective antidepressant. You should also take the person to his or her doctor, who will check to see if the symptoms are being caused by another illness or by side effects of a medication.

The AD patient's doctor may also want to prescribe a prescription antidepressant to combat the depression. There are several types of antidepressants available. Some drugs can take 6 to 12 weeks before there are real signs of improvement and most need to be continued for 6 months or more after symptoms disappear. These drugs can be helpful, although many have side effects that can aggravate the symptoms of AD, such as increased confusion, memory loss, anxiety, difficulty concentrating, or insomnia.

If the doctor prescribes antidepressants for the person with AD, you should become familiar with the possible side effects and discuss them with your pharmacist. Also, be aware of possible drug interactions—make a list of all the medications the person with AD takes and go over it with your pharmacist. It's also important that antidepressants be taken in the proper dose and on the right schedule.

It's a good idea to call the doctor if the person with AD begins to have hallucinations or delusions. A number of medical problems, such as infections, changes in diabetic conditions, anemia, or side effects of particular medications may induce hallucinations or delusions. The doctor might recommend having the person's hearing and vision checked or might prescribe antipsychotic medications to treat severe hallucinations or delusions.

————— ❧ —————

SAM-e is neither a prescription drug nor an herb, but is a synthetic replication of a compound that the body makes naturally from an amino acid found in protein-rich foods. Most authorities feel that it lifts depression as effectively as standard antidepressants. The advantage of SAM-e is that it does not cause the side effects that prescription drugs often bring. If your doctor feels the person with AD needs an antidepressant, you might ask about trying SAM-e.

—————————————

# Sexual Behaviors

What if the Alzheimer's patient engages in inappropriate sexual behavior, such as exposing genitals, groping people, or public masturbation? These behaviors are all possible, but the good news is that they are not particularly common. If you do notice sexual misbehavior, analyze it carefully. Actions that might be interpreted as sexual may, in fact, be something else. For example, if you find your loved one naked, he or she may have felt too warm or have forgotten to get dressed. Or perhaps he or she simply took off items of clothing that were too tight or uncomfortable. If public disrobing is a frequent problem, you can help prevent it by buying clothes that are difficult to remove, such as blouses that button up the back.

If the person with AD engages in public masturbation, remember that it's just another manifestation of Alzheimer's disease—it's not malicious or perverted. The affected person has probably forgotten that it's socially unacceptable to masturbate in public. It may embarrass you, but since it's one of the few pleasurable activities that the person with AD has left, it might be best to try to get the person to move to a more private area and just accept it.

Sometimes parents with Alzheimer's disease approach their children sexually, which is naturally very upsetting to the adult child. Since adult children often look like their parents looked when they were younger, the person with AD, when making a sexual overture, almost always thinks the adult child is his or her spouse. If this happens to you, try to calmly explain that you are not your mother or father.

If you are upset or angry about a sexual behavior, you may reinforce the behavior or cause the person with AD to become even more agitated. You might be able to react calmly, however, if you decide beforehand how to respond to unacceptable behaviors, so you are prepared and are not simply reacting in the moment. If you figure out when and where the behavior tends to occur and what seems to trigger it, you might be able to make changes in the environment or schedule that will eliminate the behavior or make it happen less often. As with other difficult behaviors, you can also plan

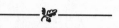

various strategies to distract and divert the attention of the person with AD.

## Sundowning and Sleep Disturbances

Sundowning, as Chapter 10 discusses, is confused, restless behavior that occurs in the late afternoon and evening. No one really seems to know why it happens, but it may have to do with the change in the light or fatigue in the patient at that time of day. Some ways to help prevent and deal with sundowning include:

- Keep activities during the late afternoon as simple as possible and even simpler after the sun sets.

- If there tends to be a lot of activity in the house in the late afternoon and early evening, it may over-stimulate the person—so try to keep her away from other activity.

- Turn on lights before the sun goes down so there isn't a great shift in the light.

- Make sure the person with AD has had enough exercise throughout the day.

- Be flexible and willing to cancel planned activities for the person with AD at the end of the day.

- Tell the person where she is and what is happening.

- If the person begins to pace, don't try to stop her—it might bring about a catastrophic outburst.

- Check with the doctor about the problem. Changing the person's medication schedule may help.

Don't dismiss the effectiveness of therapy and support groups in treating depression. Support groups help people deal with AD, learn new coping skills, and find supportive friends. Participating in a local senior center, volunteer service, or nutrition program may also help. Several "talk" therapies are quite beneficial to people with AD. One method helps people change negative thinking patterns that lead to depression, while the other type helps improve a person's relationships with others in an effort to lessen feelings of despair.

As people age, whether or not they develop Alzheimer's disease, they sleep more fitfully and tend to awaken at night more often. Alzheimer's patients may have additional sleeping problems caused by hallucinations or nightmares.

Also, the sleeping difficulties of people with AD are often caused by the disorientation and memory loss symptoms of the disease. A person with Alzheimer's might awaken at night to go to the bathroom, but then not be able to find it in the dark. Or, the affected person might get up in the middle of

———— 🦋 ————

For some men, genital exposure may not be a sexual behavior, but instead may signal the need to urinate. Agnosia, the inability to comprehend what one sees, might cause a man to urinate into a trashcan or sink because he thinks it is a toilet. Chapter 19, "Personal Hygiene at Home," offers suggestions for dealing with incontinence as well as other difficult personal hygiene problems.

the night, then forget why he is up. He might then wander throughout the house, turn on lights, and make noise, waking up the other people in the house.

What can you do to help the person with AD sleep well? Keep him active during the day. People who exercise sleep better and longer. Exercise should not be planned for the evening hours, however, because evening exercise can make getting to sleep more difficult. Also, make the person's bedroom as comfortable as possible and easy to navigate. It may help to place a night-light and even a portable toilet in the person's room.

If you have tried night-lights, portable toilets, and a good exercise regimen and the problem continues, you might want to talk to the person's doctor. He or she may prescribe a sleeping pill or sedative. The main problem with sedatives is that regular use causes side effects—such as hangover-like irritability and confusion—which aggravate the AD symptoms. Many people with AD develop a pattern of disturbed nighttime sleep and daytime naps. It might be tempting for you to encourage daytime napping because it gives you some time off during the day. In the long run, however, it is better to discourage naps so that the person with AD will sleep at night and not awaken you. You need all the sleep you can get to maintain your ability to care for your loved one with Alzheimer's.

# 12

# *How Do You Survive Stage 2?*

---

Since 1980, the number of people over 85 in this country has increased by 65 percent. For the first time in history, American families have more parents than children. And, families—or a caregiver within the family—may spend as many as 18 years caring for an elderly family member, compared to only 17 years caring for a child. A person with Alzheimer's disease may live up to 20 years with the disease. You could be in the caregiving business for a very long time.

Stage 2 of Alzheimer's brings into your life many new and difficult challenges. It is the longest stage and, in the opinion of some caregivers, the most difficult stage. As you devote more time and energy in this stage to caring for the person with Alzheimer's disease, you may experience conflicting emotions. On one hand, you love the person with Alzheimer's and may feel satisfied and even proud of the level of care you are able to provide for him or her. On the other hand, however, you may find it hard to accept the steady decline of the person for whom you are giving care. Your positive feelings may co-exist with feelings of resentment, anger, or frustration. These conflicting emotions may cause additional stress and guilt.

If it isn't easy for you to express and deal with the conflicting emotions that arise as a caregiver, you may become depressed. Or, the emotional stress you are under may manifest itself in the form of other problems, including anxiety or panic disorders. In this chapter, we'll talk about some of the emotions

———— 🌿 ————

Anxiety is the clinical name given to stress, tension, fear, or worry. It's normal to feel some anxiety almost every day, but anxiety occasionally increases to the point that it ruins your day's activities, gets in the way of enjoying life, and makes you feel emotionally paralyzed or unable to act. If that happens to you, it's definitely time to get your anxiety under control. Find a professional therapist or counselor and get help.

you might be experiencing and how to deal with them. We'll also discuss some of the potential physical consequences of being a caregiver that you should watch out for in this long second stage of the disease.

## Expressing Your Emotions

It's easy to make excuses for not talking to someone about your concerns and worries. You might feel that you are too busy to talk about your problems or that it's weak to share with others what you are going through. You should never let yourself get too busy to take care of yourself, however, and it's not at all weak to talk about your feelings. In fact, it takes strength of character to be willing to express your fears and other emotions.

There are also great benefits to expressing your feelings. If you talk about a problem to a friend, family member, teacher, or counselor, he or she might be able to help you see things in a different light. Also, simply being able to express your feelings and have someone listen may lift your emotional burden. Of course, some feelings might be harder for you to talk about than others.

### Anger

The overwhelming responsibilities of caring for a person with Alzheimer's disease may make you feel trapped and angry. In the beginning, you might not have thought it would be so difficult to be on call 24 hours a day, 7 days a week; but now, each day seems interminable. You are exhausted and isolated. As you think about your situation, you might feel tremendous anger and frustration. Or, you may not think you are angry, but then you suddenly find yourself lashing out at the person with AD or someone else who just happens to be in your line of fire. Whether you admit it to yourself or not, you are probably harboring some amount of frustration and anger. If you are having bouts of rage, you need to deal with your anger in a productive way.

If you don't deal with your anger, it may be harmful to your relationship with the person with Alzheimer's. Studies have shown that 67 percent of caregivers admit to frequently getting angry with the person with AD. About 40 percent say they occasionally lose control and shout or throw things at the person for whom they are caring. In one survey of 340 Alzheimer's caregivers, 12 percent admitted to shoving, pinching, biting, hitting, or kicking the person with AD at least once.

Anger that festers and isn't expressed may turn into uncontrollable rage that will affect every aspect of your life. Or your anger might come out in frequent frowns or snide and nasty comments, which can harm your relationships. Anger can also be expressed passively by ignoring or otherwise neglecting the person with AD and his or her proper care.

Anger that is not expressed productively will also block other positive emotions. You can't express love if you haven't already released your angry feelings. Repressed anger might also produce anxiety and fear in you. Or anger can become internalized and lead to self-destructive behaviors, such as excessive drinking or the use of habit-forming drugs. Unexpressed anger can also lead to physical symptoms—everything from frequent colds to more serious chronic illnesses.

Despite the potential dangers of unexpressed anger, anger itself is a normal emotion and one that is certainly understandable in your situation. What has happened to you and your loved one is not fair. It is tragic, and you have a right to be furious.

But how do you express your anger safely and productively? In Chapter 9, "How Do You Survive Stage 1?" we talk about joining a support group and keeping a journal. If you haven't joined a group or begun a journal, try one or both now. It's safe to talk about your angry feelings in a support group or to write about them in your journal. You might also want to visit a Web site called Alzwell Alzheimer Caregiver Page at www.alzwell.com. It offers an "Anger Wall" on which you can write your angry feelings and read those of other caregivers.

Some warning signs that your anger may be getting out of control include chronic anxiety, feeling overcommitted and overwhelmed, insomnia, feeling irritated or displeased with others, and feeling frustrated or hopeless. Other signs include sadness and depression, fatigue, and feelings of insecurity. You may also be finding it more difficult to perform your caregiving responsibilities as well as your other responsibilities in the home or on the job. If your problem is serious, you should seek professional help from a psychologist, psychiatrist, social worker, or mental health counselor. Asking for help now will help you avoid more serious problems later.

## Sadness and Grief

It's natural, of course, for you to feel tremendous sadness about what has happened to the person with AD and also to you as a result. You may feel that you have already cried and already grieved, but, in fact, grieving will be an ongoing process for as long as you are living with the disease. There is more and more to grieve as the disease progresses. You shouldn't expect to resolve your feelings of grief until some period of time after the death of your loved one with AD.

So, how do you deal with your grief and sadness? First, ask yourself if grief is a hidden part of your feelings of anger, guilt, anxiety, or depression. You may lash out at people because it's easier for you than feeling the sadness and the heartbreaking pain. If that's the case, it's time to acknowledge your grief and sadness—let yourself feel it.

You may be the type of person who doesn't think it's right to cry. If you have been the strong one in the family, you may find it easy to comfort others when they cry, but not easy to cry yourself. A good cry, however, may be one of the healthiest ways you can deal with your sadness and grief—it might prevent a tension headache or another physical consequence.

You can also manage your grief better if you are aware of the losses and problems that you can expect in the future—such as incontinence or the inability to recognize others—so that when these things happen it is not a surprise. Of course, by reading this book, you are learning what to expect.

In order to deal with your sadness and grief, be sure to take some quiet time for yourself. Also, try to find someone to talk to about your feelings of sadness, someone who can offer you comfort and support. That may be a close friend, someone from your support group, a therapist, or another family member. If a well-meaning friend responds by saying the wrong thing, ignore him or her. You will know when you have found the right person to talk to about your feelings because you will feel better afterward.

## Guilt

Guilt is one of those feelings that seem to be catching. When the person with Alzheimer's is still mentally capable, in Stage 1 and the early part of Stage 2, she may feel guilty about becoming a burden to you. Her guilt can, in turn, make you feel guilty for other reasons. As with other emotions, it's important to recognize guilty feelings and deal with them. If you don't, guilt could keep you from making clear-headed decisions about the future and doing what is right for the person with AD or the rest of your family.

What are some of the common causes of caregiver guilt? You may find yourself feeling guilty for ...

- The way you treated the person in the past.
- Being embarrassed by the person's "odd" behavior.
- Losing your temper when frustrated with the impaired person.
- Doing something you think may have made the person worse.
- Not doing something you think would have helped the person.
- Not wanting the overwhelming responsibility of taking care of the person with Alzheimer's.
- Spending time with your friends away from the person, especially when he or she is your spouse and you have been accustomed to doing most things together.
- Considering placing the person in a nursing home.

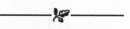

You may feel guilty because you think that the person with AD wouldn't have gotten worse if you had done something differently— taken more time with her, kept her more active, or not let her have an operation or hospital stay. If you are worried that you somehow caused or aggravated this illness, remember that Alzheimer's disease is a progressive illness and that neither you nor the entire medical profession can prevent its progression.

Some caregivers complain that the person with Alzheimer's makes them feel guilty. The Alzheimer's patient might say something like, "Promise you will never put me into a nursing home." If a statement such as this is the source of your feelings of guilt, remember that a person with Alzheimer's cannot make responsible decisions and you must ultimately make decisions for him or her. And those decisions should not be made out of guilt, but should be based on what you feel is best for you, your family, and your loved one.

Not all feelings of guilt are over big issues, like whether or not the AD patient should ever be in a nursing home. Sometimes you might feel vaguely guilty and not even know why. Or you might feel guilty about having yelled at the person with AD on a day when you were anxious or tired. If you simply say "I'm sorry," it might clear the air and make you both feel better. Also, even though you might be still feeling guilty about an incident, the person with AD—because of his or her memory loss—might have already forgotten it.

If you feel guilty about doing things for yourself and by yourself, remember that it is better for the person with AD if you take care of yourself first. If your life lacks meaning and fulfillment outside of caring for him, you are bound to take out your unhappiness in negative ways. On the other hand, if you take time to enjoy the companionship of friends and do other fun and relaxing activities, it will keep you strong and in better spirits.

As with other feelings, when guilty feelings are a problem and they keep you from making clear-headed decisions, you may find it helpful to talk with an understanding friend, family member, or someone from your support group who might be going through something similar. Learning that others have feelings of guilt may help you put your own guilt into proper perspective.

Guilt keeps you focused on the past rather than moving forward in life. It can keep you paralyzed—even though you can't change the past. You can, however, make changes in yourself so you don't repeat the action you are feeling guilty about. If you constantly snap at the person with AD and then feel guilty afterward, you can try to get more rest, more exercise, or more time away from the person so that you are less tense.

## Identify Your Trigger Points

One way to deal with anger and other emotions is to learn what seems to trigger them. The same kinds of incidents may cause you to get upset on a regular basis. Instead of allowing an angry or other stressful reaction to happen repeatedly, you can try to take control of the situation.

For example, let's say that a particular thing the Alzheimer's patient does over and over upsets you. You may get angry and yell at him or her and then feel guilty afterward. It's not likely that you can stop the AD patient from doing whatever it is, but it might help to try to understand and analyze that situation and others like it that upset you.

First, identify the feeling that is triggered by the event. Is it anger, fear, sadness, or guilt? These are all very different feelings that have different causes. Then, once you know what it is that you feel, admit that you have the feeling, even though the admission may be difficult for you. Don't try to blame others or yourself for the feeling, just accept that it is your feeling and that you want to understand it.

Then, try to analyze the feeling and what triggers it. Try to get some distance from the situation. What is it about the particular event that makes you feel this way? What does the situation mean to you? Sometimes writing about an incident that triggered strong emotions will help you understand and begin the problem-solving process. Or talk about your feelings with someone you trust—a friend or a therapist.

Once you understand your feelings and how they are triggered, you'll be able to make a plan. Figure out what you can do differently when you recognize that the feeling is returning. Make the plan very concrete. You can't just say that you will change. You have to know specifically what you will change and how.

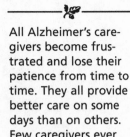

All Alzheimer's caregivers become frustrated and lose their patience from time to time. They all provide better care on some days than on others. Few caregivers ever receive the thanks they deserve. Nevertheless, they work to ensure that the person with AD is loved, nurtured, and cared for in the best possible way for many years. The legacy that this army of Alzheimer's caregivers leaves for the world is a living example both of courage and of love.

Then, when you feel the emotion being triggered again, carry out your plan. It may be to take a step back and go into the next room or to take a walk. You won't always be prepared and in control, but being aware and planning ahead can help to reduce the emotional stress of any kind of repetitive and upsetting situation.

## Love

And, finally, what about your positive emotions? What about love? You are probably a caregiver because of your love for the person with AD. It hurts to see your loved one suffer. He might be your parent or your spouse or partner. You care about him very much, and you know that if the situation were reversed and you had Alzheimer's disease, he would do the same for you.

Despite the love you feel, however, you soon realize that caregiving can be a difficult, exhausting, and thankless job. It requires everything you have. You are a cook, housekeeper, and nurse all rolled into one. You have to eat when the person you are caring for eats, sleep when he or she sleeps, and do everything else whenever you can find a minute.

As the disease progresses, you may get little thanks from the person with Alzheimer's disease. The affected person must struggle to make sense out of her limited world and may become less and less aware of you and your needs. You won't get praise or gratitude from the person with AD, and probably not from anyone else either. How do you maintain the love you once felt for the person when she is so different now? How can you continue to be loving when you are exhausted from all the work of caregiving?

There are no easy answers to those questions. For most caregivers, having other sources of friendship, love, and pleasure in their lives besides the person with AD is very important. Ultimately, however, you will have to find the answers inside yourself. In their book, *The Best Friends Approach to Alzheimer's Care*, Virginia Bell and David Troxel (Health Professions Press, 1996) suggest an approach to follow that can help you maintain your love and respect for the person with AD. Here are some of their key suggestions:

- Treat the person as an adult, not as a child.
- Take the person's feelings seriously.
- Take the person's interests, history, and heritage seriously.
- Be a best friend—have empathy for the person and show affection frequently.
- Laugh together frequently.
- Be flexible.
- Be nonjudgmental—of the person with AD and of yourself.

# Physical Reactions

By Stage 2 of Alzheimer's disease, you may have been taking care of the person with Alzheimer's for a number of years. Even if you felt strong and capable at the beginning, by now, if you haven't taken excellent care of yourself, you could have compromised your immune system, leaving you more susceptible to fatigue and infections or viruses that cause illness.

## Fatigue

As Chapter 11, "Dealing with Difficult Behavior," discusses, sleep disturbances become common as Alzheimer's disease progresses. When the AD patient can't sleep, it often affects your sleep. You may also simply not have enough hours in the day to get a good night's sleep, or you may not be able to fall asleep because of anxiety about your numerous responsibilities. When you regularly don't get enough rest, you are likely to either get sick or get depressed. What are some ways you can avoid fatigue?

First, make sure that you deal with the Alzheimer's patient's sleep problems. They are not something you can ignore if they keep you from getting enough rest. If the person with AD gets up and quietly sits on the sofa at night, you don't need to get up and try to get her back to bed. If she is noisy and awakens you, however, you need to find a way to help your loved one sleep through the night.

---

### One Caregiver's Journey

"The funniest thing that happened to my mother while she was still living in the senior residence gave everyone in the place a great laugh. I went to visit her one day and walked into the lobby, which was full of residents who often sit there throughout the day. People called out to me, 'Congratulations! Congratulations!' 'What for?' I asked. One of them said, 'Your mother got married last night.' 'Married?' I was stunned.

"I went upstairs and there, as always, was Leonard in the apartment with my mother. I said, 'Mother, I hear you got married last night.' She looked at me and said, 'I did?' I looked at Leonard. He beamed—it was true. I found out the name of the rabbi who had performed the marriage and called him, upset that he had married my mother and Leonard in their condition. The rabbi was very apologetic. He said that he had led the usual Saturday service at the residence the previous weekend, and that Leonard had approached him with my mother, saying they wanted to be married.

"Most people would have known if they talked to my mother that something was wrong, but Leonard was still in pretty good shape, and he did all the talking. Since most of the people in this residence didn't have Alzheimer's, the rabbi thought this was a very romantic thing. He waived the blood test and other state requirements, in view of their ages, and married them. I told the rabbi that if he registered the marriage with the state, my mother would lose her Social Security. He said he realized his mistake now and wouldn't do that. He later had that reinforced because Leonard kept calling him saying he couldn't find the marriage license. The rabbi sent him two more and he still couldn't find them!"

---

There are also things you can do during the day to keep yourself from getting exhausted. It's important, for example, to allow the person with Alzheimer's to do as much as possible and only provide help when she needs it. Sometimes it's hard to watch the person with AD do things when you know you could do the same thing faster and easier. When a person with Alzheimer's does all or part of her own personal care, however, it helps maintain her strength, self-esteem, and independence. And even having the few minutes to do something else will help you.

Remember to exercise, eat well, and plan time for relaxing activities. Sometimes you can exercise and relax with the person with AD. At other times, it's best to find ways to relax on your own.

## Stress-Related Illness

The stress of being a primary caregiver for a person with Alzheimer's may cause you to become ill yourself. Physical symptoms, including headaches, stomachaches, backaches, frequent colds, or even more serious conditions can develop when you don't take care of yourself, don't eat right, don't exercise, or don't express your feelings productively.

If you are discouraged and tired, you are likely to get sick more often. When you get sick, it only compounds the problems you already have. Who takes care of the person with AD when you are down with the flu?

So how do you stay healthy? It may sound like a broken record to you by now, but the answer is the same: Eat well, exercise, get enough rest, express your feelings productively, get help, and take time off. Don't abuse alcohol. Don't smoke or use lots of caffeine. Don't over-medicate yourself, and get regular check-ups from you doctor. If you take good care of yourself and don't let yourself down—you won't let your loved one down either.

Numerous studies confirm that some form of support is beneficial for caregivers who are at risk for depression, anxiety, sleep disorders, and other problems. Therapy has been shown to be a particularly effective treatment for depression. Eighty percent of people with depression improve when they receive treatments of medication, therapy, or the combination of

In general, Alzheimer's caregivers, compared with noncaregivers, report more health problems and take longer to recover from them. One study that confirmed this looked at the effectiveness of the flu vaccine in 64 older men and women, half of whom were caring for partners with AD. Vaccines stimulate the immune system to produce antibodies, which are part of the body's defense against infections and viruses. In the noncaregivers, the flu shot stimulated the increase in antibodies as it was expected to, but among the Alzheimer's caregivers, only 37 percent produced an adequate antibody response. This demonstrated that the immune systems of the AD caregivers were more impaired than those of the noncaregivers.

both. Those who receive both therapy and an antidepressant drug are much less likely to experience a recurrence of depression over a three-year period than those who receive medication only. Another study showed that individual and family counseling plus support group participation by caregiving spouses delayed institutionalization of patients with Alzheimer's by almost a year. In yet another study, targeted behavioral therapy techniques improved the quality of caregivers' sleep.

## When Is It Time to Get Help?

One of the hardest aspects of your role as a caregiver is realizing and accepting that you might need help for the emotional strain of being a caregiver. Your worry, anxiety, or emotional pain may be affecting your sleep, your eating habits, and your relationships with everyone, including the person with AD. Your ability to function in your daily life may be increasingly affected by the stress you are under.

At first, you may seek out family or friends. After a while, however, talking to family or friends may not make you feel any better. Even the most well-meaning friend might not be able to help you deal with some of the deep emotional issues that may have been triggered by your role as an Alzheimer's caregiver.

Caring for someone over a sustained period of time is much more emotionally and physically draining than sporadic, short-term care. It's important, therefore, to have the support of people who can empathize with you and share in your experiences.

Therapy, in particular, can help you address the underlying causes for your emotional distress. It can help to restore your emotional well-being, and help you learn about yourself and grow from the experience of being a caregiver. The very fact that you feel safe enough to talk about your feelings, your conflicts, and your frustrations will allow you to make lasting, positive changes in your life. And, particularly at a time when you are gradually losing your long emotional, trusting relationship with the person with AD, a therapist may provide an important new source of trust.

If you live in a large city, it might be a good idea to ask the local Alzheimer's Association for a referral to a therapist. The therapists they recommend are likely to have training or experience in treating caregivers of Alzheimer's patients. Although it isn't essential that the therapist you choose have experience with the disease, he or she should at least have helped others in similar circumstances.

Another alternative is a therapy group run by a private therapist. In some cities, such as Los Angeles, Alzheimer's support groups are led by therapists, but in other areas AD caregiver support groups may not have a therapist as a facilitator. Hopefully, you will seek out the help you need in whatever form seems best for you. But whatever you do, don't stay isolated. Don't try to tough it out alone. You may be strong, but even you can use the love, support, and wisdom of others through this ordeal.

### One Caregiver's Journey

"It's hard enough to be an AD caregiver when the person doesn't live with you, as in my case. But when you do have to take care of an Alzheimer's patient at home, the only way to survive is to develop some kind of life of your own. Going to support groups is one of the best things you can do because everybody there knows what is going on. Many caregivers in my group were very isolated before they came because their families were no help. And people they thought were friends were generally friends for a particular thing like playing tennis or going to the theater, which they didn't have as much time for anymore. Very few people hang around and are there for the caregiver. That's why I really believe in the value of Alzheimer's support groups."

## Avoiding Isolation

What can you do to avoid isolation? Even though you feel exhausted and down, it's important to try to make new friends or keep up with old ones. Make time for yourself away from the person with AD to spend with old friends. Make new friends by participating in activities you enjoy. If you like playing cards or going to baseball games, don't give up these activities because you are too busy. Also, become involved in new activities—like an Alzheimer's support group—in which you will meet people with whom you have things in common.

Whatever you do, don't just sit at home and feel sorry for yourself. Go to places where things are happening. Even a trip to the mall might help lift your spirits. Offer your services in neighborhood or volunteer organizations. Stay involved in the world and with the people around you. Yes, you have the hardest job in the world, but you can't let it take every minute of your time.

# 13

# What to Expect in Stage 3

---

Stage 3 of Alzheimer's, the final stage of the disease, is perhaps the most heartrendingly brutal. By Stage 3, 50 percent of the affected person's brain will have been destroyed by the disease. Both mental and physical deterioration will become so severe in this stage that the affected person will, ultimately, be completely dependent on you or on professional caregivers.

Stage 3 usually lasts from one to three years, although the rate of deterioration can be much longer or much shorter, depending upon the individual. The younger a person is when he or she is diagnosed with Alzheimer's, the faster the disease generally progresses. As with the earlier stages of the disease, not everyone will progress at the same rate or display the same symptoms in Stage 3.

———— ✣ ————

Since he or she will require total physical care during Stage 3, families face the difficult decision of whether and when to place the Alzheimer's patient in a nursing home. Don't wait for a crisis to make the decision that your loved one would be better off in a home. Allow enough time to find the best facility for the patient. (See Chapters 21 and 22 for information on when to make the decision and how to choose a facility.)

# Severe Intellectual Impairment

In Stage 3, the AD patient's intellectual impairment is obvious all of the time. An affected person often won't recognize his wife and children, or he may confuse his children with his parents. He may not be able to comprehend a simple request or complete a relatively easy task. He may not be able to remember what you say to him for longer than a few minutes, if he even understands you. This increasing impairment affects speech, comprehension, and all other cognitive or intellectual functions.

*One Caregiver's Journey*

"My mother was a wonderful grandmother, and she and my daughter had been very close. When my daughter had a child, she naturally wanted my mother to see her new baby. Even though my mother was pretty far along with Alzheimer's, my daughter hoped that my mother, who liked babies, would understand that this baby was her great-grandchild. I told my daughter that my mother would probably not understand who the baby was, but she was still hopeful. When we went over to visit, my mother held the baby and played with her, but she had no idea who the baby was. It was very disappointing to my daughter."

## Severe Speech Impairment

As Stage 3 begins and progresses, the AD patient will usually experience a steady decline in the ability to communicate verbally. Depending on the individual, the person may completely lose all speech ability or may retain some verbal ability until the end of his or her life.

The progression of the loss of speech in Stage 3 will vary among individuals, but in general, you might observe several steps of speech loss. First, there might be an increase in repetitious questions or statements. As the disease progresses further, a person with AD may substitute more similar-sounding words for words he cannot recall, making his speech difficult to understand. "Real" might be used instead of "feel," or "tree" instead of "tea." After that, the person may begin to make up words or speak in gibberish. Then, his or her vocabulary may become limited to dozen or fewer intelligible words. Finally, the person might only be able to say a single word or two.

As the disease progresses even further, the person with AD may not be able to communicate with words at all. He or she may groan, scream, or make grunting sounds in an effort to communicate. At the same time, he or she may be losing comprehension and may not be able to understand most of what you say. At this point, however, even though the person may not understand the words you say, he or she may still be able to respond to the emotion in your tone of voice.

## Very Little Awareness of Surroundings

In addition to verbal communication, by the third stage of AD, the person with Alzheimer's will have very little awareness of the people and the environment around him. He will not recognize most other people—even close family members and even himself in the mirror.

The affected person will also be completely disoriented as to time and place. He won't have a clue where he is or what day, month, or year it is—or even whether it is night or day. He may also continue to have visual and auditory hallucinations, which will contribute to his inability to realize where he is and with whom he is speaking.

## Loss of Other Mental Functions

Other intellectual functions that are severely impaired at this stage include judgment and the ability to solve problems. The person with AD may eat spoiled, bad-smelling food or even the dog's food. He may put everything in his mouth or try to touch everything. No longer able to connect smoke with the danger of fire, he may refuse to leave a smoke-filled room.

In Stage 3, wandering becomes much less of a problem because, as the disease continues to destroy the memory and other intellectual abilities, the person with AD will normally

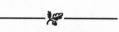

Even though she has lost the cognitive skills that our society values highly, an Alzheimer's patient can still do things that will improve the quality of her life. She can still enjoy listening to music, playing with a pet, or spending some time outdoors. Even though she will not be able to remember or speak about the experience later, she will still have enjoyed the moment.

———————— 🌿 ————————

As the devastation of Alzheimer's disease moves through the brain, it attacks parts of the brain that correspond to the person's symptoms. The first nerves to die are generally in the hippocampus, a part of the brain that is important for learning and memory. The destruction then moves to the temporal and parietal lobes, which control language and other cognitive functions. Once this area is affected, the person may hallucinate, suffer seizures, and lose the ability to speak, to read, and to recognize places, objects, and faces. Finally, the cortex begins to be destroyed, which controls many behaviors including interpreting sensory information, intellectual abilities, emotional expression, and physical movements.

become more and more lethargic. She won't spontaneously initiate activities but will spend most of the time sitting in a chair or lying in bed and will appear uninterested in what is going on around her. It's not surprising that this is the case since the person with Alzheimer's has lost most of her ability to take part in daily life.

In Stage 3, the person with AD will generally not have as many emotional outbursts as she may have had in Stage 2. After a certain point, the Alzheimer's patient will express little or no emotion—although she may still respond positively to your expression of love or affection. Sadly, some people even lose their ability to smile.

In Stage 3, you can expect your loved one's mental impairment to be so severe that she will eventually be …

- Unable to speak or be able to communicate verbally with only a very limited vocabulary.
- Unable to understand most of what others say.
- Unable to recognize others.
- Unaware of surroundings.
- Unable to do crafts or exercises.
- Unaware of dangers in the environment.
- Generally apathetic and lethargic.
- Unable to express emotions.

## Refusal to Eat

As Alzheimer's disease progresses into Stage 3, it is common for an affected person to lose his appetite. He may refuse to eat or may eat very little. The affected person is likely to lose both the interest in food and the physical ability to eat without assistance. Caregivers may need to prepare special diets for late-stage AD patients. Some people with AD may go on eating binges or express a desire for sweets, but that is more likely to happen in Stage 2. By Stage 3, most AD patients have little interest in food and often refuse to eat.

The person with AD may not want to eat for several reasons. Sometimes he simply may not remember that eating can take away the feeling of hunger. He may have a dry mouth from all the medications he is taking. The disease may cause changes in his sense of smell and taste. The affected person may not eat because he believes he has already eaten or because he becomes confused and forgets what he is doing. Or, he may be constipated or depressed, both of which suppress the appetite. Unfortunately, because of his impaired speech, he can't talk to you or a professional caregiver about these problems.

By Stage 3, most people with AD also have difficulties using silverware, a problem that may have developed in Stage 2. At a certain point, if you are still the affected person's primary caregiver, you will have to feed him. At this time, patients also begin to have difficulty swallowing, which naturally contributes to the eating problems. The difficulty swallowing may be because the person doesn't remember how to swallow or because brain damage has impaired the swallowing reflex. It may be necessary to cut out certain foods that are difficult to eat and replace them with easier-to-swallow and higher-calorie foods. See Chapter 18, "Mealtime Traumas," for help dealing with all aspects of the difficulty of eating.

Even if you are able to make sure the person receives good nutrition and a good diet, he or she is also likely to lose weight during Stage 3, simply as a consequence of the disease.

> When swallowing becomes difficult for a person with AD, there is a danger of choking. The affected person should be in an upright position during and for at least thirty minutes after a meal. Also, because of the danger of choking, be sure that you, if you are alone with the person, know how to perform the Heimlich maneuver (or that someone nearby does if you are in a nursing facility).

## Complete Dependency

In addition to the difficulty communicating and the problems with eating, other physical and mental disabilities develop in Stage 3 that will make the AD patient entirely dependent on caregivers. In Stage 2, you may have tried to let the person with AD do as much as he or she could do independently, but by Stage 3, that will no longer be possible.

An Alzheimer's patient may have trouble controlling her bowel and bladder, either because of infections or blockage,

─────── ❧ ───────

Although AD patients in Stage 3 lose much of their ability to communicate, they still respond to touch, facial expressions, and tone of voice. While understanding very few words, a person with AD may still appreciate your expressions of warmth and concern. Some people with AD may still be able to sing along with music or at least enjoy music. Although the losses you are witnessing are devastating, it helps to focus on the abilities and personality traits still left.

─────────────────

or simply because she forgets the location of the bathroom. An AD patient's loss of coordination also becomes more obvious in Stage 3. She may develop generalized muscular rigidity and eventually may not be able to walk or stand without help. As these difficulties progress, she may want to just sit quietly rather than try to undertake the increasingly stressful demands of daily living.

Many patients in the later stages of AD may require hospitalization at some point. As they become less mobile, they are more prone to secondary medical problems, such as pneumonia and skin ulcerations. Chapter 14, "Medical Care Issues in Stage 3," gives more information on these problems.

### One Caregiver's Journey

"I didn't want my mother to have to move out of her senior residence, so a couple of years before I had to place her in a facility, I hired a woman to be with her all day. My mother had recently become incontinent, but she wouldn't wear diapers. The woman who took care of her tried to get her to change her underwear so it wouldn't smell, but she wouldn't do that either. That was the one thing that she was absolutely adamant about and is the reason I had to eventually move her into a nursing facility. The people in the residence complained that she smelled, but she adamantly refused to wear diapers."

## Incontinence

One of the symptoms of Alzheimer's disease that most people don't like to talk about or even think about are the bowel and bladder accidents that occur in the later stages of the disease. These problems are very common, however. Some people with AD may develop urinary incontinence in Stage 2, but by Stage 3 most patients will have trouble controlling bodily functions. Why is incontinence such a problem?

The person with AD may not remember what the sensations mean and thus is unaware of the need to relieve herself. Or the person may no longer remember that this feeling means that she needs to go to the bathroom. If she does remember that the sensation means it's time to go to the bathroom, then memory problems and perceptual difficulties may make it difficult for her to find the bathroom. At night, it might be even more difficult for her to locate the bathroom.

If incontinence develops while you are still caring for the person with AD in your home, see Chapter 19, "Personal Hygiene at Home," for suggestions on how to deal with the problem. There are several medical reasons for urinary incontinence and, even in the late stages of the disease, the cause can sometimes be identified and treated.

## Inability to Perform Most Activities Without Help

By Stage 3 of Alzheimer's disease, an affected person is also likely to experience an increased loss of basic motor skills. She may be unsteady, may trip or fall frequently, and may have difficulty even sitting and holding up her head. She will need help bathing, dressing, eating, and using the bathroom. It may seem as though her brain is no longer able to tell her body what to do.

The loss of mobility and lack of coordination that occurs with the disease affects both large and small movements and many areas of life. Some of the common problems or symptoms you will notice in Stage 3 include the following:

- Poor balance
- Stooped posture
- Unsteadiness, frequent stumbling or falling
- Difficulty getting up from a chair
- The inability to walk or stand without help
- The inability to bathe or dress without assistance
- General muscle weakness
- Muscle jerking or tremors
- Long periods of sitting
- Little or no response to stimuli
- Long periods of lying curled up in bed

In AD patients, every instance of incontinence is not necessarily related to Alzheimer's disease. Since incontinence affects the quality of life of the patient, when it occurs, it should not be denied or ignored, but talked about and, if possible, treated. Your doctor should be consulted about the problem to see if he or she can identify a treatable condition that might be causing the incontinence.

---
🦋
---

Some people with Alzheimer's disease may exhibit tremors or shaking similar to Parkinson's disease. Parkinson's can coexist with Alzheimer's, and it may be difficult to differentiate between the two conditions when Alzheimer's is in the advanced stages. Nevertheless, a person with AD should be evaluated by a doctor when tremors, shaking, or rapid jerking movements of the limbs or the body occur. Treatable conditions, such as anxiety or a side effect of medication, could be the cause.

---

- Constant rocking or other repetitive motions
- Difficulty swallowing
- Possible seizures
- The tendency to sleep more
- Possible grabbing or kicking
- Blankly stares into space
- The inability to perform most purposeful movements
- The inability to cope with basic needs

You should speak with a doctor as soon as any of these conditions begin to occur frequently. Muscle stiffness or even muscle jerking and tremors are examples of symptoms that could be caused by the patient's medications, instead of AD. Adjustments in the medication could then reverse the symptom. By the time Alzheimer's disease interferes with the person's ability to walk, talk, or swallow, serious medical conditions such as pneumonia can develop.

## The Final Months

Sadly, by the time a person with AD reaches the later stages of the disease, he may no longer be recognizable as the person he once was. He will have lost most of his personality, his ability to communicate, to understand others, to move around, to control his bowel or bladder, or to eat on his own. He may seem like an entirely different person than the one you once loved. He is dying, but he may live on in this condition for many months.

How can you deal with this heartbreaking process? You can focus on the abilities of the person that remain—the sense of touch, hearing, and the ability to understand and sometimes even respond to the emotion in your tone of voice and demeanor. Touch him in gentle, affectionate ways and tell him that you love him. Although you may not hear an "I love you, too," you will give him enormous comfort in that moment.

# 14

# *Medical Care Issues in Stage 3*

---

A person in the last stage of Alzheimer's disease may suffer from a variety of medical problems that can be caused by the disease, aggravated by the disease, caused by side effects of medications, or simply a result of the person's age and increasing frailty. These problems can be serious and life-threatening or they can be problems that make the person with AD uncomfortable, thus reducing his or her quality of life.

Unlike other older people who may experience some of the same medical problems, a person with AD will usually not be able to tell you or a professional caregiver about the pain or symptoms he or she is experiencing. Therefore, you should know what kinds of medical problems are common in the last stage of AD so you can make sure that your loved one is getting the best possible care.

—————— ❧ ——————

A person with AD might fall because he or she cannot accurately judge the height of steps, curbs, and door thresholds. To help prevent falls, the edges of steps can be made more visible by highlighting them with brightly colored tape or paint. Or, when you can't lock doors to stairways, you can place high barriers in front of them to prevent the person with AD from using the stairs. See Chapter 17, "Securing Your Home," for more on this issue.

*One Caregiver's Journey*

"My mother developed a prolapsed rectum fairly late in the disease. I took her to a proctologist who wanted to do surgery. I was afraid to let her have the operation because when an Alzheimer's patient has surgery, the effect of the anesthesia can cause the AD symptoms to get worse. So, I kept putting it off, but finally I had it done. I asked the doctor to be sure that they didn't give her too much anesthesia. He said they would make it as light as possible. It turned out okay. I didn't notice any big difference afterward."

# Falls

As people get very old and frail, the risk of falls and injuries from falls increases. One third of older adults who live at home fall and injure themselves each year. A person with AD, however, is at an even greater risk for falls and subsequent injuries as the disease progresses than most older people. You should know the cause of falls in older people generally and AD patients specifically, as well as the things you can do to help prevent falls.

An older person might have other medical conditions that make him unsteady and make walking difficult. Arthritis, Parkinson's disease, foot problems, visual impairment, and inner-ear problems causing loss of equilibrium or dizziness when getting up are among the health conditions that affect walking or balance and increase the risk of falling. Diabetes can affect sensation in the feet, making it hard for the person to know that his foot has touched the ground.

Reaction time also slows down in older people, and their balance is often less reliable. Older adults in nursing homes may get very little physical activity and therefore become weak and out of shape, which also increases the chances of a fall. Stiffening of the joints as a side effect of medication or from Alzheimer's disease itself can also make walking more difficult and increase the likelihood of falls. The effects of blood pressure medications, water pills, tranquilizers or sedatives, and some antidepressants and antihistamines may increase the risk of a fall.

In addition to medical conditions that can affect all older people, AD patients have additional problems that place them at an even higher risk of falling. Brain cell deterioration with AD causes an even slower reaction time than that of most older people. Poor depth perception or trouble with visual-spatial relations—both common with AD patients—can result in misinterpreting the environment and prevent the person from seeing something in front of him.

People with AD often develop apraxia, or loss of coordination (see Chapter 10, "What to Expect in Stage 2"). Apraxia can affect all sorts of purposeful movements, including walking. In addition, memory loss from the disease can cause the person to forget a cane, walker, or other walking aid or forget how to use it correctly. A further complication with Alzheimer's disease is the decreased judgment of the person, which might cause her to take unnecessary risks.

Despite the fact that many falls are caused by medical problems or AD itself, an equal number of falls are preventable. Many falls are caused by poor environmental factors such as bad lighting, loose carpeting, slippery floors, or cluttered surroundings. To decrease the possibility of falls, the person's environment—whether that is your home or a nursing home—should be made as safe as possible.

If the AD patient is still at home, make sure the lighting is good, that there are grab rails for her to hold on to, that she has comfortable and supportive shoes, and that there are clear, uncluttered walking paths throughout the house. See Chapter 17 for more on how to prevent falls and accidents in the home.

Healthcare facilities should also do all that they can to prevent falls, even though it isn't realistic to expect that a person with AD will never fall. See Chapter 22, "How to Choose the Right Nursing Home," for general considerations regarding a facility's safety policies. Some of the things you should expect from a facility to keep your loved one as safe as possible include:

If you have any concerns about the possibility of a fall by a loved one in a nursing home, discuss them with the staff. You may have suggestions that the staff of the facility would be happy to implement. If they are not willing to listen to your concerns and consider your ideas, you might need to move your loved one to another facility.

———————🌿———————

If your loved one is in a nursing facility that uses restraints, you should question that policy or find another facility. Research suggests that restraints may not prevent falls. They should thus be an option of last resort and never used solely for the convenience of the caregivers. Drugs or chemical restraints can cause harmful interactions with existing medications. Physical restraints can cause health problems, such as incontinence, pressure sores, depression, increased agitation, and deterioration in the person's overall condition.

- The rooms and areas where residents walk are safe and uncluttered.
- The floors are not waxed or slippery.
- The residents are engaged in regular walks and exercise.
- Doctors and physical and/or occupational therapists are available to consult with patients about mobility issues.
- All falls are thoroughly investigated.
- The staff is willing to discuss your concerns.
- All reasonable steps are taken to decrease the patient's risk of falling.

## Pressure Sores

Pressure sores (also called decubitus ulcers) develop when a person is bedridden for prolonged periods. In persons who are not yet bedridden, tight clothing or long periods of sitting in the same place can also cause pressure sores. The skin of older people is often very fragile and thin due to both aging and inadequate nutrition. An AD patient's refusal to eat or difficulty eating may result in malnutrition and weight loss. When the person with AD loses fat tissue, bony areas such as those around the heels, hips, elbows, shoulders, shoulder blades, spine, knees, buttocks, and ankles are particularly at risk for pressure sores.

In addition to pressure sores, when the person's skin is extremely fragile, bruises and cuts can develop even from routine bathing. You can tell when a person is developing pressure sores if you notice red spots or bruises anywhere, but particularly in the areas of the hips, tailbone, heels, or elbows.

Prevention of pressure sores is particularly important because once the skin is damaged, it is very difficult for it to heal. If the person with AD is still mobile, make sure that he does not sit for long periods in the same place. Since any kind of exercise is good for the affected person, make sure that he gets up and moves around on a regular basis.

If the person with AD is no longer able to walk on his own and must either lie in bed or sit in a chair, develop a schedule for changing his position at least once every two hours. Turning relieves pressure on bony areas and allows the blood circulation to return to the tissue in the area. The person must be turned very gently, however. If he is dragged across the bed, the friction could easily damage the skin.

To further protect the person with AD from painful pressure sores, there are various types of mattresses and devices that can help protect his fragile skin. Hospitals often use foam mattresses or beds that move automatically, both of which are helpful. Medical supply houses sell air cushions, water cushions, gel pads, foam pads, heel pads, elbow pads, and other types of devices that can protect particularly vulnerable areas. These aids should be used in addition to—not instead of— frequently turning the patient.

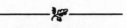

If you are caring for a person with AD in your home, have a nurse or home health-care worker show you how to prevent pressure sores. In general, pillows can help ease the pressure. When a patient is lying on his back, place a small pillow under his lower leg so that his heels don't rest directly on the mattress. Also place pillows between his knees and ankles to prevent them from touching each other.

## Dental Problems

In the late stages of the disease, it is very important that you or the nursing home caregivers be responsible for your loved one's oral hygiene. If the affected person's teeth and gums are neglected, it can lead to painful infections. Teeth can decay and gums can become irritated and inflamed, resulting in pain, bleeding, and ultimately systemic infections.

Sometimes an Alzheimer's patient's refusal to eat is caused by ulcers or infections in the mouth that caregivers have not noticed and that the person is not able to tell them about. The person with AD should have regular checkups with a dentist and, if there seems to be a problem eating, a dentist or dental hygienist should immediately examine him or her.

Both those with natural teeth and those with dentures need to have proper oral care. For patients with their own teeth, caregivers will have to brush the teeth and floss the gums. For those with dentures, caregivers will have to clean both the soft tissues of the mouth and the dentures.

If your loved one resists going to the dentist or refuses to let the dentist look in his or her mouth, try to find a dentist who works with older people. Some dentists are more effective with people with dementia because they work more slowly and gently. Also, if the dentist suggests a general anesthetic during dental care, remember that the anesthetic could have a harmful effect on the AD patient and should only be used if absolutely necessary.

# Vision and Hearing Problems

Older people often have problems with their eyes. Many are afflicted with diseases that reduce vision, including glaucoma, cataracts, and macular degeneration. These diseases can cause an older person to think that she sees something that is not really there. Problems with vision can also cause an older person to fall more often. Since, in the late stages of the disease, an Alzheimer's patient may not be able to describe the problems that she is experiencing, it is important that caregivers are aware of potential problems with vision.

Visual problems are particularly troublesome for people with Alzheimer's disease, who are already confused due to memory loss. Not only must glasses prescriptions be checked regularly, but when you suspect problems with vision, it's also important to make sure that the person with AD has her eyes checked by an ophthalmologist, a medical doctor who specializes in eyes, who will check for various diseases.

Older people also frequently have hearing loss. Hearing trouble complicates things further for those with AD, who are already confused, so it is important to correct hearing loss if at all possible. An audiologist and a doctor should be able to perform tests to distinguish between comprehension problems due to AD and actual hearing loss that can be corrected with a hearing aid.

One problem with hearing aids is that they amplify background noises, which may confuse or agitate a person with AD. To help the situation, try to reduce background noises and speak directly to the person. Also, the person with AD usually cannot manipulate the hearing aid to control the volume or squeaking. He may find it irritating and take it out and misplace it—something that also frequently happens with glasses and dentures.

# Dehydration

Dehydration may occasionally be a problem for people in the earlier stages of AD, but for those in the later stages of the disease it is a common and often serious problem. Dehydration causes fatigue, apathy, constipation, and abdominal discomfort. Severe dehydration can be fatal. The amount of fluids each person needs to prevent dehydration varies by the individual and by other factors, such as the time of year. Certain conditions may lead to dehydration, including vomiting, diarrhea or diabetes. Some medications, such as diuretics or heart medicine may cause dehydration.

The common symptoms of dehydration include the following:

- Thirst
- Dry mouth
- Refusal to drink
- Fever
- Rapid pulse
- Dizziness or lightheadedness
- Confusion and hallucinations
- Fatigue
- Apathy
- Constipation

If you are unsure about whether or not your loved one is getting enough fluids or is dehydrated, check with his doctor.

## Constipation

Constipation is another medical problem that often affects older people and can be a particular problem for those with Alzheimer's disease. This is not something that either caregivers or patients like to talk about, but it is important medically to monitor and prevent constipation in patients. Constipation causes discomfort and distress and, unless treated, can lead to other problems, such as fecal impaction—hard feces that block the rectum—and fecal incontinence.

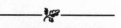

Make sure you get the Alzheimer's patient's eyes checked regularly. As people age, the curvature of the cornea becomes less smooth and more irregular, causing many people to need glasses for astigmatism. Many older people who may be nearsighted or farsighted already wear glasses, but they may also need their prescriptions checked since it may no longer be adequate. Or, if the person wears contacts, he may no longer be able to handle them and will need glasses.

Problems with constipation don't usually arise until the later stages of AD, but they could occur earlier. With many persons with AD, simply setting up a regular schedule of taking the patient to the bathroom can help. This usually works best about 30 minutes after breakfast, when the person is likely to need to make a bowel movement.

Other methods of preventing constipation include making sure that the person's diet includes whole fiber, such as whole-grain breads, cereals, vegetables, and fruits. These foods should be given to the person with AD every day. Also, he should be as active as possible, since physical activity helps to facilitate bowel movements. Make sure the person walks at least twice a day. If the person is confined to his bed, it may help to turn him every two hours and to help him sit up in a chair for part of the day, if at all possible. Increasing the amount of fluids the person with AD drinks will also help prevent constipation. The patient should be encouraged to drink water throughout the day. In the morning, hot tea, coffee, or prune juice may also help stimulate a bowel movement.

If the person with AD is constipated despite activity, fluids, and a high-fiber diet and has gone for more than three days without a bowel movement, he may have to use a laxative. Do not give him a laxative, however, without consulting his doctor. All laxatives have side effects and unless used carefully, they can lead to serious problems in older people, such as fecal incontinence or intestinal obstruction.

There are several kinds of laxatives. Bulk-forming laxatives are fiber-based mixtures that take from 24 hours to three days to work. They may cause dehydration unless taken with plenty of fluids throughout the day. Salt-based laxatives work more quickly, but can cause cramping, diarrhea, and dehydration. Lubricants, such as mineral oil, can be dangerous for people who have difficulty swallowing and can also interfere with the absorption of certain vitamins. Other types of laxatives may be recommended for temporary relief, but are not helpful in chronic cases. In every case, check with the person's doctor before using a laxative, because all have side effects and may be harmful if taken regularly or if the patient has other problems, such as diabetes.

## Infections and Pneumonia

A bedridden person with advanced Alzheimer's disease is very vulnerable to infections, such as influenza or pneumonia. In fact, people with AD generally die of illnesses that are common in people confined to bed—including pneumonia, urinary tract infections, malnutrition, and dehydration. Even the flu could be fatal in a weak, bedridden AD patient. To help prevent these infections, the person with AD should receive flu and pneumonia vaccines each year. As we have stressed elsewhere, a good diet, plenty of fluids, and some form of mild exercise will also help prevent infections.

*One Caregiver's Journey*

"Once, my mother developed pneumonia, and I took her to the hospital. She wouldn't get undressed at the hospital and the staff unfortunately didn't understand Alzheimer's disease. They argued with her and tried to force her to undress. I called the man who ran the nursing facility where she lived, who was a wonderful man. He came to the hospital, but the hospital staff tried to get him out of her room. I insisted that they let him stay because he was the only one who could deal with her. Finally, when they couldn't get her to cooperate, they let us get her undressed."

No matter how careful you or your loved one's professional caregivers are, there will come a day when death is very near. How prepared will you be? The next chapter covers some of the issues that arise as your loved one nears death.

# 15

## *Before Death Comes*

---

Death is not an easy topic to think about. If you are the caregiver of a person with Alzheimer's disease, however, it's a reality you must eventually face. Alzheimer's is incurable and terminal. Unlike other terminal illnesses in which there is often a relatively short period of time from diagnosis until death, the person with AD may live up to 20 years after diagnosis. And, by the time the patient is in the final stage of the disease, if not before, you must face the issues surrounding her imminent death.

If a patient reaches the final stage of the disease, Alzheimer's will be the actual cause of death, although there will also be an immediate cause of death. With AD patients, the immediate cause of death is usually a complication, such as pneumonia, dehydration, infection, or malnutrition, which arises from the deterioration of the entire system caused by Alzheimer's. Some patients with Alzheimer's disease may die earlier from other terminal illnesses, such as stroke, heart attack, cancer, or other causes and thus may not reach the final stage of AD.

*One Caregiver's Journey*

"A man in my group was taking care of his wife at home, with nurses helping him around the clock. His wife was 90, in the late stage of AD, and had been bedridden for a very long time. She didn't know anyone, couldn't talk, and really couldn't do anything. One day, the nurse said that she thought his wife had pneumonia and insisted that he call 911. He did, and his wife was immediately taken to the hospital. The pneumonia was cured and she came back home.

"A lot of people don't know that when you call 911, you give up control. They must revive by doing everything they can. I suggested that he talk to his children and have a plan for what they will do the next time there is an emergency. If the family decides that they want to revive her no matter what, that's fine. If they decide not to take extraordinary measures to revive her, that's fine, too. Since his nurse insisted that he call 911, he also needed to find staff who would support his decision if it was otherwise."

## Medical Intervention

Hopefully, you began to plan for the last stage of AD and made decisions about how to handle some of the medical intervention issues that you will face at the end of your loved one's life while he or she was still able to participate in the discussions (see Chapter 6, "Plans for the Future"). At that time the patient may have given you an Advance Health Care Directive or a Durable Power of Attorney for healthcare.

If you have been given the power to make healthcare decisions for the Alzheimer's patient, what are the decisions you will be faced with in the final stage of AD? We all want to die with dignity and in as comfortable a manner as possible. How do you make sure that the person with AD has the best possible quality of life until the very end? How do you make decisions about what medical interventions should be used?

If the person with AD, when she was still able to, told you whether or not she wanted extraordinary measures taken to prolong her life, her wishes should be respected in making your decisions. If the person with AD has not given you guidance, you will have to make decisions on your own or consult with your doctor and with other family members about what to do.

There are no right or wrong decisions regarding medical interventions at the end of life. When a patient reaches the final stage of Alzheimer's disease, many doctors and families choose to provide comfort measures only. Others want to do all that is medically possible to keep the person alive. If you are not certain about what to do, it may help to learn more about the kind of measures that are taken to prolong life.

## Feeding Tubes

Eating difficulties often occur in the late stage of Alzheimer's disease, as discussed in Chapter 14, "Medical Care Issues in Stage 3." Various types of devices can be used to feed and/or provide the patient with fluids. The doctor might want to use an IV (an intravenous infusion line), which would generally be hooked up to the patient's arm or a feeding tube that is connected directly to the stomach.

When the person with AD is not near death and is not completely incapacitated, feeding and hydration tubes should always be used. If the only function of the tubes, however, is to prolong the dying process, using them is not necessarily the best treatment, and doing so may actually make the patient suffer more. Nevertheless, feeding tubes are often used because the medical staff at the facility or hospital does not want to appear to be negligent or because the family is unwilling or unable to make a decision that would allow the person to die.

If you decide that it's best not to use feeding tubes, the person with AD will die of dehydration or starvation. Is that a painful way to die? Most clinical evidence shows that death by dehydration is actually a compassionate and comfortable way to die. Losing interest in eating and drinking is part of the natural dying process, so when you don't feed or provide fluid to a dying person who doesn't want food or drink, it isn't

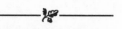

It's tough to watch a loved one die and not offer food or drink. To do so, however, may be more for your own benefit than it is for your loved one's. Both family caregivers and professionals dislike feeling helpless and usually have difficulty doing nothing. Keeping busy also prevents us from having to feel our grief. Soothing words and reassuring physical contact, however, may ultimately be more compassionate and better for the dying person than food or drink.

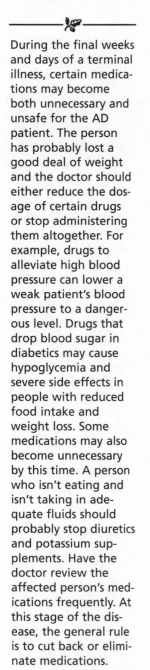

During the final weeks and days of a terminal illness, certain medications may become both unnecessary and unsafe for the AD patient. The person has probably lost a good deal of weight and the doctor should either reduce the dosage of certain drugs or stop administering them altogether. For example, drugs to alleviate high blood pressure can lower a weak patient's blood pressure to a dangerous level. Drugs that drop blood sugar in diabetics may cause hypoglycemia and severe side effects in people with reduced food intake and weight loss. Some medications may also become unnecessary by this time. A person who isn't eating and isn't taking in adequate fluids should probably stop diuretics and potassium supplements. Have the doctor review the affected person's medications frequently. At this stage of the disease, the general rule is to cut back or eliminate medications.

starvation as we usually define it. It certainly isn't the same as withholding food or fluids from a healthy person who is hungry or thirsty.

On the other hand, hydrating the person with a feeding tube or IV will prolong the dying process and might make the person more uncomfortable than he or she already is. The tubes themselves might be unpleasant or they might fill the person's body with fluids that could then gather in the throat and lungs. Also, a person with AD might be confused and frightened by the feeding tubes.

Not using feeding tubes does not mean that the person with AD is getting inferior medical care, nor will it make him or her suffer more. In fact, the person may die more comfortably without feeding tubes than with them. Nevertheless, you should get competent medical and legal advice before you make a decision to forego using feeding tubes. And you should, of course, always respect the wishes of the dying person.

## Medication

At the end of life, medication—such as antibiotics for pneumonia—can be an extraordinary measure. You may choose to forego treating your loved one with antibiotics for pneumonia because it will only prolong the dying process and will certainly not cure the underlying problem, which is Alzheimer's disease. As with feeding tubes, it's important that you make the decision of whether or not to allow the doctor to treat the AD patient with antibiotics very carefully. If you do not treat it, the pneumonia will very likely be fatal. If you do treat it, however, you may be simply prolonging life—and not necessarily for your loved one's benefit.

What about pain medication? If the person with AD has a disease such as cancer that is causing pain, he or she will need a pain medication, such as morphine. As the disease that causes pain progresses, the amount of morphine or other narcotic required to control the pain increases.

The goal of pain medication is to keep the affected person as comfortable as possible. If the person has difficulty swallowing, you or a nurse can administer liquid medication by mouth, or use rectal suppositories. Pain can also be relieved by morphine that's put under the tongue and absorbed through the membranes of the person's mouth or by special adhesive patches containing opiates, which can be absorbed through the person's skin.

## Surgery

In some cases, the doctor of a person in the third stage of AD may recommend surgery for any of a number of conditions. Should you consent to surgery for the AD patient at this late stage in the disease? In general, that depends on the capabilities of the person. If he or she is still walking and able to carry on some activities of daily life, you might want to consider it, bearing in mind that the effects of the anesthesia may cause further confusion and mental deterioration in the patient. It might be wise to get more than one medical opinion before consenting to the surgery.

If the person is already bedridden and near the end of life, it is unlikely that most doctors would recommend surgery. If it is recommended, you may not want to consent to it, although again, a second medical opinion might help you make the decision.

## Resuscitation

Cardiopulmonary resuscitation, or CPR, a means of reviving a person after the heart has stopped, is less effective on frail elderly patients—such as those in the late stage of Alzheimer's disease—than it is on younger, healthier victims of such traumas as accidents or heart attacks. The small percentage of elderly patients who do survive CPR are often in worse condition than before their hearts stopped, and may have to spend their last days, weeks, or months in a hospital ICU.

Because CPR cannot provide long-term survival for a person in the final stage of AD and will not improve his or her

In most states, the law prevents euthanasia, which is the act of ending the life—by lethal injection or some other method—of an individual suffering from a terminal illness or incurable condition. The decision to withhold extraordinary medical treatment and let nature take its course, however, is generally accepted both legally and ethically. Patients (or their designated representatives) have the right to refuse life-extending treatment. If you are unsure of your legal rights in this area, contact an attorney.

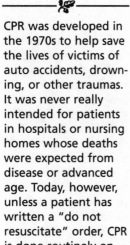

CPR was developed in the 1970s to help save the lives of victims of auto accidents, drowning, or other traumas. It was never really intended for patients in hospitals or nursing homes whose deaths were expected from disease or advanced age. Today, however, unless a patient has written a "do not resuscitate" order, CPR is done routinely on every patient whose heart stops—whether in a hospital or a nursing home or on the street.

quality of life, but in fact may diminish it, it is often best to have a "do not resuscitate" (DNR) order placed on the patient's medical chart. Having such an order does not mean that you are giving up on the life of your loved one. It only means that you do not want to prolong his or her life by using aggressive medical treatment.

As dementia progresses to a point at which the health and abilities of the patient have deteriorated so that she is unable to walk or do other purposeful movements, has difficulty swallowing food or refuses to eat, has infections, such as pneumonia or urinary tract infections, has very limited speech, if any, and has other symptoms, the decision not to use medical technologies except to provide comfort care for the patient certainly becomes a reasonable one.

Ultimately, the affected person's quality of life is the most important consideration. If you decide that the goal in the care of your loved one is comfort and emotional well-being, rather than artificially prolonging his or her life, that should be your guide in making decisions about medical treatments.

## Where Will the Patient Die?

As death nears in the last stage of AD, you will have to decide where the patient should die. If the person with AD is already living in a nursing home and you are happy with the care and the facility's end-of-life policies, it is certainly best to leave the person there. If the person has been transferred to a hospital for some reason, you should make your wishes known about the use of aggressive medical interventions as discussed earlier.

If you have been taking care of a person with Alzheimer's in your home, it may be beyond your capabilities to provide total bedside care in the final stage of the disease. To keep the person at home, you may want to have full-time nursing care assistance, if you can afford it. Another alternative that many doctors and family caregivers of Alzheimer's patients use is hospice care, which is available through Medicare.

Hospice care is a program designed for patients who cannot be cured. It can be provided either in your home or at a special hospice facility—in about 90 percent of cases it is provided in the home. The purpose of hospice care is to help the affected person make the most of each remaining day of his or her life by providing comfort and relief from pain.

Medicare requires that hospice patients be certified by a doctor as being terminally ill and with a life expectancy of six months or less. Medicare beneficiaries who choose hospice care no longer receive treatment toward a cure, but do receive close medical and supportive care from a hospice, including a variety of services not otherwise covered by Medicare.

If you choose hospice care, a plan-of-care will be established by the AD patient's doctor and the Medicare-approved hospice team. Under this plan, Medicare will cover such aspects of care as …

- Doctor's services.
- Intermittent nursing care with 24-hour on-call care.
- Medical appliances and supplies related to the terminal illness.
- Outpatient drugs for symptom management and pain relief.
- Short-term acute inpatient care, including respite care, home health aide, and homemaker services.
- Physical therapy and occupational therapy.
- Medical social services.
- Counseling, including dietary and spiritual counseling.

You can find out more about hospice programs from the National Hospice and Palliative Care Organization online at www.nhpco.org or Hospice Net at www.hospicenet.org.

## The Last Moments

How will you know when your loved one's death is near? There are signs that precede death in most people, as body systems slow down and finally cease to function. For some

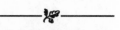

End-of-life decisions generally involve deciding when is the right time to let go. If the goal of treatment at this stage is keeping the patient comfortable, rather than prolonging life, then caregivers should attempt to provide whatever forms of pleasure and comfort are possible and resist interventions that diminish comfort. Simple things like the touch of a hand or soothing words will offer greater comfort than feeding tubes or breathing machines.

For many people, it's important to be present at the exact moment of death but, of course, that is not always possible. If you can be there not only at the exact time of death, but also in the days prior to a loved one's death, you can help to ease the way for the dying person. Being there in the final days and final moments can be one of the most moving and meaningful experiences of your life.

people, the signs will appear a few hours before death and for others, a few days. There is no particular order in which these signs occur, and some people do not experience all of them.

If you know what to expect when your loved one is dying, it may be easier for you to be calm and continue to give him or her loving support. Also, remember that there are no right or wrong ways to behave at the time of your loved one's death. You may simply want to be with him and assure him that you are there. On the other hand, if you cry or feel afraid, it is all right. The death of a loved one is frightening and heartbreaking, and it's okay to experience your feelings.

What are the signs that the affected person is near death? First, he will show less interest in eating and drinking. For many patients, refusing to eat is an indication that he is ready to die. A person may only want enough fluids to keep his mouth from feeling too dry. As the caregiver, you should offer, but not force, food and drink.

The person's urinary output may decrease in both amount and frequency because of his decreased fluid intake as well as a decrease in circulation through the kidneys. There is nothing you should do about this, unless the affected person wants to urinate, but cannot. Then, discuss the problem with a nurse.

As the body weakens further and the patient begins to detach from the environment more, he may spend an increasing amount of time sleeping. The person may appear to be uncommunicative, unresponsive, difficult to arouse, withdrawn or in a comatose-like state. These are normal symptoms as the person detaches from his surroundings and begins to let go. These signs are partly due to changes in the metabolism of the body. You should simply let him sleep.

The person's regular breathing pattern may change as he nears death. Breathing may become irregular with short 20- to 30-second periods of not breathing at all. Different breathing patterns are caused by a decrease in circulation in the person's internal organs. He may appear to be working very hard to breathe and may make a moaning sound with each breath.

This sound doesn't usually mean the person is in pain, but is simply the sound of air passing over relaxed vocal cords. As the time of death gets even closer, breathing may again become regular, but shallower and more mechanical-sounding. The person may also experience periods of rapid but shallow breathing. Sometimes you can help the patient to breathe more easily if you prop him up slightly in bed.

As the oxygen supply to the brain decreases, the patient may become restless or have disturbing dreams. It's not unusual for patients to pull at bed linens, to have visual hallucinations, or even to try to get out of bed at this point. It will help if you reassure him in a calm voice that you are there.

The dying person's hands and arms, feet and then legs may be increasingly cool to the touch. At the same time, the color of the skin may change. These are both indications that the blood circulation to the body's extremities is decreasing and is being reserved for the vital organs. The patient may feel hot one minute and cold the next as the body loses its ability to control its temperature. You can provide or remove blankets as needed and sponge him with a cool washcloth if it seems to help. If it will make the patient more comfortable, you can also change wet garments or bed linens.

Loss of control of bladder and bowel function may also occur around the time of death. You can protect the mattress with a plastic sheet or put a waterproof padding under the patient and change it as needed to keep him comfortable.

Secretions may collect in the back of the dying person's throat, causing rattles or gurgles when the patient breathes through his mouth. He may also cough up mucous and possibly start to choke or vomit. Try to keep the air in the room humid by using a cool mist vaporizer. It also might help to place the affected person on his side and to use swabs dipped in cool water to relieve the dryness in his mouth.

When a person reaches the last stage of dying, the body will begin its final process of shutting down. At that time, all of the physical systems will stop functioning—breathing will cease, the heart will stop beating, the eyelids may be partially open

Near the end of an Alzheimer's patient's life, you may feel upset if he refuses your attempts to make him more comfortable. Despite the fact that you have spent years taking care of him, at this point, it is more important to simply be with him than to try to do things for him. Also, since hearing is the last of the senses to go, assume that he will be able to hear what you say in his presence.

People don't die as dramatically in the real world as they do in the movies. There's nothing otherworldly about the transition from dying to death. Even with the best preparation, the moment of death may come as somewhat of a shock to you. But you will get through it. Your fears are always worse than reality, and your ability to cope will be greater than you might expect.

with the eyes in a fixed stare, the mouth may fall open slightly as the jaw relaxes, and any waste matter in the bladder or rectum will be released as the sphincter muscles relax. When the patient cannot be aroused and all of these major vital functions stop, death has occurred.

# After-Death Decisions

Before your loved one's death, you should have decided on a mortuary or funeral home, so that you will know what to do with the body at the time of death. Since the costs of funerals are very high, you might be able to save money by doing research in advance of the person's death. The funeral will also involve a number of decisions, many of which you may want to make before your loved one's death, so you are not faced with everything at that upsetting and overwhelming moment.

## Should There Be an Autopsy?

The only way to definitively tell whether or not your loved one actually had Alzheimer's disease and not some other form of dementia is to conduct an autopsy of his or her brain after death. If your loved one had expressed a desire for an autopsy or you want a definitive diagnosis or want to donate his or her brain to an Alzheimer's disease research center for study, it's generally wise to make those arrangements in advance, although it can be done at the time of death. You can contact the Alzheimer's Association or Alzheimer's Disease Education and Research (see Appendix C) to learn more about autopsies and research centers.

Autopsies can be expensive, but if the person's brain is also donated for research, the cost may be absorbed by the research institution. An autopsy and a donation of the person's brain to research can further our knowledge of Alzheimer's disease, so it's definitely something to consider. And contrary to what many people think, a brain autopsy will not prohibit any type of funeral you wish to plan.

## What Type of Funeral?

You will have to make many choices regarding what type of funeral or service to have after your loved one's death. Do you want a religious service? A memorial service? Do you want a traditional ground burial or would you prefer to have your loved one's body in a mausoleum? Do you want to cremate the body? If so, what do you plan to do with the ashes?

Many of these issues may be traditional in your family. You may already have purchased funeral plots, for example, or your family can always use a local funeral home. You may have already discussed your loved one's wishes when she was well or you can have to make all of the decisions yourself. In any case, it's often helpful to have someone who has known you or the family throughout the course of the disease—a friend, a rabbi, a priest, a minister, or a healthcare professional—help you plan the funeral.

# 16

## How Do You Survive Stage 3?

───────────── ❧ ─────────────

Dealing with the death of someone you love is not unique to the family and caregivers of those with Alzheimer's disease. We all lose those we love at some point. Alzheimer's disease, however, has caused the affected person to change dramatically from who he or she once was—a kind of death of the person before his or her actual death. This complicates the grieving process for you as an Alzheimer's caregiver. You might grieve throughout the course of the disease, and death is just one more traumatic change—the last one.

There are other issues that will affect the grieving process for you. As the caregiver of a person with AD, you have devoted a good portion of your time and your emotional and physical energy to caring for your loved one. Now, he or she is gone. How do you pick up the pieces of your life—professionally, practically, and emotionally?

*One Caregiver's Journey*

"Leonard was so happy with my mother. He once said to me about his case manager, 'What do I need her for? There are only two women I need in my life. Your mother and you.' He was so sweet. Months passed in the new marriage until one day, my mother went down for her regular three meals without Leonard. They sent someone upstairs to check on him. He was in bed and had died in his sleep. They called me and I went over, worried about how this would affect my mother. When I got there, she was sitting on the couch in her living room. Two policemen and a coroner were there. She didn't know who they were, but was not at all disturbed by the commotion. I told her that Leonard had died. 'Who's Leonard?' she asked. I suppose she never really knew who he was. After Leonard's death, she didn't appear to notice his absence. When I mentioned his name or showed her pictures I had taken of the two of them, she looked at me blankly."

## Are You Ready to Let Go?

You have had to let go of your loved one with AD in many ways throughout the course of the disease. You have had to let go of the things you loved about her—her conversation, her sexual interest in you, her wit and humor, as well as her recognition of you.

You have even had to let go of your caregiver role little by little as she got sicker. You may have had to place her in a nursing home or you may have had to turn over her care to nurses or other professional caregivers in your home. Now, however, you must let go completely of both your loved one and your role as caregiver.

Because you have already had to let go of many aspects of your loved one, you may know when and how to let go better than caregivers of other terminal patients. Nevertheless, even though you have had to gradually let go for years, don't expect that completely letting go of your loved one will be easy. Allow yourself the time and space to grieve properly.

Letting go of the role of caregiver may also be harder than you think. For many people, the role of caregiver becomes a primary source of self-validation. When the person you are caring for dies and you no longer have a role, it may affect your self-esteem. You may feel lost, worthless, or useless without the responsibility of taking care of the person with AD.

If you feel any of these feelings, don't allow them to turn into depression or despair. You are worthwhile, even if you no longer have the person with AD to care for. You must deal with your feelings and go on to find new ways to fill your life with meaning.

## There's Nothing Wrong with Feeling Relief

A long-term illness, particularly one that goes on for many years as does Alzheimer's, may leave the caregiver and family with mixed feelings. As you watch someone you love suffer the gradual loss of his mental capabilities and then reach the stage in which he cannot even get out of bed, you may wish that he could be out of his misery. When he actually dies, you may feel relieved—both that it's over for your loved one and that it's over for you.

You may experience guilt or shame for "wishing it were over" or for seeing your loved one as already "gone" intellectually. The feeling of relief at the death of a person with AD, however, is normal. There is no need to feel guilty for being relieved that the person has died. Death is a natural part of life and it must come to all of us at some point. If you wanted the final stage of AD to be over, it was only because it was painful for you to watch your loved one lose more and more of his abilities. If you felt relief after the death of your loved one, it was because you did not want him to have to suffer anymore or because you saw that his life was so limited at the end and that the inevitable was so near.

If you discuss feelings of relief with family members, close friends, your caregiver support group, or a mental health professional, you will understand that your feelings are normal and you shouldn't feel guilty about them. And you shouldn't feel guilty about wanting to go on with your own life now, after neglecting many of your needs for so long.

*One Caregiver's Journey*

"My mother just stopped eating, and I didn't want to have her fed with an IV. I think that by the time an AD patient dies, it's a relief. The caregiver and family can no longer remember her as she once was and, of course, she doesn't know most of the family. My mother knew me because she saw me so much, but she didn't know anyone else. She didn't know my brother or my children."

## Guilt, Anger, and Depression

After your loved one's death, you may have many feelings that will come and go for months and even years. The feelings initially will include shock and denial, then sadness, grief, guilt and anger. With Alzheimer's disease, the shock and denial stage of loss may have come many years before—probably at the time of diagnosis. The emotions that may be most present in the final stage of the disease are guilt and anger and, of course, sadness and grief.

It's important that you feel all of your feelings at this time. Your feelings may also include hostility, fearfulness, apathy, self-doubt, and emptiness. You may feel depressed, angry at the deceased for dying, unable to concentrate, and extremely sad. Bereavement may also cause you to be, at least temporarily, more closed off from others, and thus may affect your other relationships.

### Guilt

Caregiver guilt at this stage of Alzheimer's disease often arises from the feeling that you should have done more for the person with AD. Caregivers frequently remember things that could have been done for the person who died, but weren't done for one reason or another. This type of realistic guilt is common. Rather than focusing on what you didn't do for the person with AD, however, try instead to focus on all the things you were able to do for him or her.

Sometimes, a caregiver will feel guilty about a situation they could do nothing about—which is irrational guilt. Both types of guilt must be dealt with because unresolved guilt can be harmful, both physically and mentally.

We often think we are feeling guilt, when what we are really feeling is grief or sadness. For example, the tough decision to institutionalize the person with AD may make us feel guilty. But, in reality, if you made that decision it means that your loved one was getting sicker or more debilitated. Instead of feeling guilty, the emotion beneath the guilt was sadness—sadness that you are now facing the imminent death of your loved one. Also, by turning over the care of the person to others and not actually being there on a day-to-day basis, it only heightens the feelings of grief and sadness. If you are not in touch with your grief and sadness, however, you may experience it as guilt.

## Anger and Depression

Some caregivers don't feel guilty, but instead look for someone else to blame. You may feel anger toward the doctor, nurses, or other people surrounding the person with AD or anyone you think could have done something differently and somehow could have made it better for him or her. Even if these feelings are ultimately proven to be irrational, it's better to express them to a tolerant and sympathetic listener. In reality, what you are angry about might not have made much of a difference. Rather than suppressing your anger, find a safe and healthy way to express it. Anger, whether it is rational or irrational, is a normal, healthy part of the grieving process.

Your anger and frustration may lead to depression. You may start to feel weary and exhausted and want to sleep a lot. You may feel that no one really understands your feelings, and it's

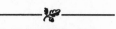

It isn't helpful when people tell you not to feel guilty about a difficult choice, such as putting your loved one in a facility. Of course you feel guilty—you did something you didn't want to do, even though you felt you must. What's important, however, is what you are really feeling beneath the guilt—frustration, loss, grief, and anger. If you can express those feelings instead of guilt, you will probably get the support and comfort you deserve.

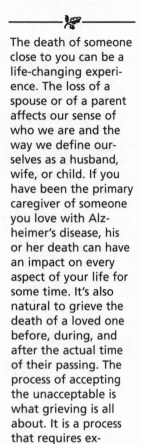

The death of someone close to you can be a life-changing experience. The loss of a spouse or of a parent affects our sense of who we are and the way we define ourselves as a husband, wife, or child. If you have been the primary caregiver of someone you love with Alzheimer's disease, his or her death can have an impact on every aspect of your life for some time. It's also natural to grieve the death of a loved one before, during, and after the actual time of their passing. The process of accepting the unacceptable is what grieving is all about. It is a process that requires extremely hard work over a period of many painful months or years.

best to just suffer in silence. You may also not feel like socializing. Don't let these feelings lead to depression. Make yourself get involved in activities and see other people. Your participation in life will help prevent and relieve feelings of depression.

If your despair continues and gets deeper, contact someone who will listen, preferably a professional counselor or a member of the clergy. If depression still persists, a doctor or psychiatrist might prescribe antidepressant drugs to help alleviate your feelings of depression and hopelessness.

## Experiencing Sadness and Grief

Despite other feelings you may experience in the final stage of the disease and at the time of death, grief and sadness are primary. These feelings of loss are a natural and important part of life. It's not a sign of weakness to feel sad, but rather a healthy response—and evidence of the love you feel for the person you have lost. As an Alzheimer's caregiver, you have to mourn both the physical loss of your loved one with AD and also what might have been or what you feel should have been had he or she not had the disease. As you mourn any death, you also have to face your own mortality, perhaps for the first time in your life.

Learning to feel and experience your sadness and grief is a necessary part of being a caregiver—and of being human. Unless you recognize and experience your grief and give yourself time to mourn, it may turn into anger, depression, helplessness, or abandonment. Although the grieving process is different for each person, there are stages of grief and common experiences.

### Anticipatory Grief

Since Alzheimer's disease is a prolonged illness characterized by serious memory impairment, family members usually begin grieving the loss of the person's "former self" long before the time of death. This is sometimes referred to as anticipatory grief, and it can be just as painful as the grief one feels at the actual time of death. Ultimately, however, antici-patory grief is a way of allowing us to prepare emotionally for the inevitable. When you know someone is dying, you can seek out the support of other family members, spiritual advi-sors, and friends.

Most people with Alzheimer's disease do not die suddenly, although incidents such as a fatal accident, a heart attack, or suicide can certainly happen to a person with AD. A death that happens unexpectedly generates shock and confusion for the loved ones left behind. Unlike anticipatory grief, this type of loss can leave you perplexed and searching for answers. If a sudden death occurs, give yourself plenty of time to grieve and get as much support as possible from others.

## Symptoms and Stages of Grief

Any type of grief can cause both physical and emotional symptoms. Physical symptoms include heart palpitations, tightness in the throat, shortness of breath, sweating, and dizziness. Other physical symptoms that might occur during the grieving process are upset stomach, headaches, sleep and appetite disturbances, and lack of energy. You also might be more susceptible to illness and might have nightmares or dreams about the deceased person.

Emotional symptoms of grief include trouble with memory, feeling distracted or preoccupied, bouts of irritability and anger, depression, and passive resignation. If you have experi-enced a loss and are hurting, you may feel that your emotional responses are unreasonable, that the death of your loved one was a long time coming and you should just accept it. It's important not to judge yourself too harshly, however, and to give yourself the space to experience your feelings. Our grief often surprises us and fills us with emotions that may be un-expected or overwhelming.

It's crucial that you take care of yourself during this period of bereavement by maintaining a proper diet and getting enough exercise and rest. Even if you don't feel like taking care of yourself, you should—because taking care of your body can help heal your mind and your broken heart.

Grief is sometimes divided into stages. Some stages of grief may be revisited many times as you go through the grieving process. The stages usually include:

- Bargaining—trying to prevent the inevitable
- Shock and denial at the time of the loss, coupled with the inability to return to usual activities
- Anger or rage about the loss
- Sadness, depression, loneliness, and a sense of isolation
- Acceptance and finally adjusting life to the reality of the loss

Most people who have lost someone close to them go through all or some of these stages, although not necessarily in this order.

## Coping Strategies

Some people cope best when they take time for quiet reflection. Others do better when they fill their time with exercise or other activities and distractions. Some people may deal with their grief by engaging in reckless or self-destructive activities, such as excessive drinking. Some may visit the gravesite a lot, and others not at all. Some may want to write in a journal, draw, paint, or express feelings in other creative ways, while others would never think of doing those kinds of things. Some people might want to go to favorite places they shared with the person, and others might want to avoid those places.

Although some forms of coping may be healthier than others, it's important to let yourself heal in your own way. There is really no right or wrong way to deal with a loss. You might do something that seems odd to others, but it might be healing for you. Don't let others make you feel that you need to heal in a particular manner.

As a coping strategy, many people find it helpful to seek out either other people dealing with a loss or trusted friends. It's very important to get support while you are grieving in order to regain some sense of control and to work through your feelings. A trained counselor, a support group, or a friend can help you sort through feelings such as anxiety, loss, anger, guilt, and sadness.

## How Long Does Grieving Last?

Although grief affects each person differently, recent research has shown that intense grieving lasts from three months to a year after a loss and many people continue experiencing profound grief for two years or more. The grieving process depends on the individual's belief system, religion, life experiences, and the type of loss suffered. Prolonged bereavement is not unusual.

Sometimes people who love you will want you to stop grieving. They may indicate that it's been a long time since the loss and you should stop feeling sad. That may cause you to feel that there is something wrong with you or that you are behaving abnormally. That's not true, however. Healing from a significant loss just takes as long as it takes.

Grief is a process, not an event. Your loss isn't something that you get over—it's a process of acceptance that you go through. By consciously going through the grieving process, you can develop personal strengths to cope with other types of loss and difficulties that may come later in life. Acceptance of the loss means gaining a perspective—a new sense of self and what you can do with you life.

Finally, here's some general advice for going through the grieving process:

- Let yourself feel!
- Give yourself quiet time alone.
- Think about who you were before the loss and who you will be after the grieving process.
- Be as open as you can be in expressing all of your feelings.
- Cry when you need to.
- Express any anger or sense of unfairness you feel.
- Tell someone you trust the story of your loss.

Although there are many ways you can grieve, you have to be careful that you aren't doing things to avoid dealing with grief or sadness. For example, you might be avoiding your emotions through excessive activity or by using alcohol or other drugs to mask your grief. If you don't let yourself grieve, you may act out in other ways, such as being resentful toward those who try to help you. Ultimately, avoiding grief will only prolong your agony.

———— 🪶 ————

If you are a religious or spiritual person, you may question your faith in God, in yourself, in others, or in life while you are grieving. Many people experience a temporary paralysis of the spirit, express anger or outrage at God, or feel cut off from God and their own souls. If that is your experience, you should know that it's not uncommon. A member of the clergy or spiritual advisor can help you examine the feelings you are experiencing.

- Find ways to say good-bye.
- Don't be hard on yourself.
- Don't drug yourself.
- Take life one day at a time.
- Don't make major decisions while you are grieving.
- Don't withdraw or run away.

Although you should never rush your grieving process, if feelings of being overwhelmed with grief continue over a long period of time, you should consider seeking professional support. You may find it too difficult to move through your grief on your own or only with the help of family and friends. A professional counselor can help you explore and resolve some issues in a confidential atmosphere and in ways that friends and family can't.

## Moving On

When your loved one with AD dies, you may feel afraid of what lies ahead for you. As a caregiver, you committed yourself totally to the care of the Alzheimer's patient. You may have moved in with him or her or moved the person to your own home. You may have given up your job, your own independence and even your family and friends. You may have become so involved with the care of the affected person that you really removed yourself from normal day-to-day living. Your entire life may have been focused on comforting and making the person with AD feel safe and loved.

Then your loved one died, and now you are left to try to find your way back into the world. A feeling of emptiness may occur after the funeral as supportive friends and family members return to their own activities. Feelings of loneliness, isolation, and depression may also become more intense at that time. You might feel that no one has ever suffered as much as you have. For some people, that lonely feeling will lift suddenly. For others, it may take months to move to the next phase of grief.

As you finally begin to emerge from your grieving process, how do you start to live again? There is really no single answer to that question. Each person has to find his or her way back into the world. It's not an easy process. There is, however, life after caregiving, and you will find meaningful new activities if you look for them.

You have to be willing to start over and find new opportunities—renew old friendships or make new ones, find a job that you feel good doing, do volunteer work, find a new hobby, or revive an old one. The important thing is not what you do, but that you do something that brings you back into the world. As you begin to participate in activities, your mood will brighten, and life will begin to take on a new perspective.

It may help to realize that the person you loved who died of Alzheimer's—before he or she lost the capability to understand—would have wanted you to adjust to life again after his or her death. The stage of moving on may take time—it's part of the grieving process. But as you move on and resolve your grief, thinking about the past and planning for the future will both become easier and easier.

## If You Are Not the Primary Caregiver

If the person with Alzheimer's was close to you—for example, your father—but your mother was the primary caregiver, how can you help her at the time of his death? You will certainly have your own grief to deal with, but your surviving parent may need your help as well. How can we help others who are grieving?

The following suggestions may help you provide support for those close to you who are grieving:

- Be available.
- Listen without giving advice.
- Allow him or her to cry and feel the pain.
- Don't force the grieving person to share feelings if he or she doesn't want to.
- Give physical comfort through hugs and gentle touches.

- Don't be afraid to mention the deceased person—the grieving person is likely to be already thinking about him or her.
- Realize that no one can replace or undo the loss.
- Be there later, when other people have all gone back to their routines.
- Offer practical help around the house.

If a grieving person comes to you with a lot of anger to express, patiently allow him or her to get it all out—including the anger or bitterness he or she may feel toward the person with AD, against other family members, or against God. Anger is a normal part of the process of grieving, and a way we try to find meaning in what has happened.

# 17

# *Securing Your Home*

───────────────❦───────────────

It's never too early to make changes to your home that will make it safe for your loved one with Alzheimer's disease. As you have seen, as AD progresses, the affected person is likely to experience not only memory loss, but also loss of coordination and visual difficulties, all of which can lead to falls and other injuries. Even though it may seem that the person with AD can navigate the home environment easily, increased difficulty could come at any time. It's best to begin to secure the home as soon after diagnosis as possible.

Modifying your home to make it safer for the person with AD does not have to be a major renovation project. Your goal should be to only make modifications that are necessary, to keep them simple, and to balance your needs against those of the person with Alzheimer's. You can make adaptations that modify and simplify your home without severely disrupting your household, and can purchase most of the gadgets and supplies necessary for home safety at stores that carry hardware, electronics, medical supplies, and children's items. If you can't install the items yourself, find a reliable handyman to help.

—————— ❦ ——————

As you secure your home, set aside an area for yourself to relax undisturbed—a respite zone—that is off-limits to others. We all need private time, and for care-givers, it's crucial. The respite zone could be your bedroom, home office, or a place in the attic or basement. Wherever it is, it should be your private place that is arranged the way you want it. Without a respite zone, you will risk burnout from the heavy burden of care-giving.

# General Safety Considerations

Your first job in making your home safe is to go through it carefully and look for potential hazards. What kinds of things are hazards to people with AD? Things that might not bother a person without dementia can be very confusing and even dangerous to people with Alzheimer's disease. Appliances, furniture, and lighting fixtures that were once familiar to the person with AD can, when his or her abilities become compromised by the disease, be the cause of harmful accidents.

# Is It Too Cluttered, Busy, or Noisy?

Clutter is a problem for people with AD in different stages of the disease. In the early to middle stages of AD, clutter may be a problem because the person with AD might hide things, and in a cluttered house it's far more difficult to find lost items. Later in the disease, cluttered areas may confuse and upset the person with AD and actually cause him to fall or otherwise harm himself.

You need to train yourself to behave differently than you always have. You need to get rid of knickknacks that are easily knocked over or fragile items that may break if the person falls or leans against them. You need to throw away piles of papers and magazines that may be distracting or disorienting to the person—and train yourself to dispose of them regularly. You need to throw out old broken or unused things that are in piles or corners around the house.

Put the clutter that you just can't bear to part with in a room or closet that you can lock. Whenever you can't decide whether or not to let go of something, either just throw it out or put it in a locked closet or room. Don't leave it lying around while you are thinking about it. It's particularly important to keep all walkways free of clutter.

In addition to clutter, certain kinds of wall and floor coverings may be more difficult for the person with AD to deal with than others. Does your home have busy patterns on the walls, floor coverings, upholstery, or draperies? These busy designs may confuse the person with AD and cause accidents.

Too much noise in the environment can also be a real problem for the person with AD. Loud or constant noises—such as an air conditioner or furnace starting up, washer, dryer, or dishwasher noise, neighbors arguing, dogs barking, constant noise from the television or radio, buzzing from fluorescent lights, lots of shouting or conversations, traffic noises, construction noises—might disturb the person with AD.

## Is It Too Dark?

Proper lighting is a very important part of improving safety in the home. Older people tend to need much more light than younger people and people with AD particularly need lighting that helps them see obstacles in rooms. Dark corners can look like caves or holes to people with Alzheimer's disease. By reducing the dark areas in your home, you will help the person with AD get around easier and will eliminate misperceptions that might trigger hallucinations or falls.

Here are some general guidelines you can use for lighting in your home.

- Use natural lighting during the day—open curtains and other window coverings.
- Position lamps and light sources in a way that will prevent shadows.
- Light hallways, stairs, and bathrooms at night with night-lights.
- Make sure there is a light near each doorway.
- Use nonglare bulbs in all areas.
- Make sure the outside lighting is adequate.
- Make sure all rooms have adequate lighting.

## Is It Too Hot?

One reason a person with AD may become unwilling to bathe or shower is because he fears getting burned by the hot water. People with Alzheimer's are at risk for burns because they may become less sensitive to heat and cold or may not react quickly enough to prevent burns. To help prevent scalding with hot water, you should lower the temperature on the

AD patients often want to rummage through drawers and then hide various items. Since you will be locking away many dangerous things that the person should not have access to, it's a good idea to also create drawers, boxes, cabinets, or closets that are safe places in which he or she can rummage or hide things. You can get rid of safe clutter—junk mail, old magazines, old keys, buttons, or other small items—by putting them in containers that you don't mind the person with AD going through. Make the cabinets and drawers that are okay for rummaging more accessible and colorful than the ones that are off-limits. If hiding valuable things is still a real problem, some caregivers install surveillance cameras to help them locate the AD patient's favorite hiding places.

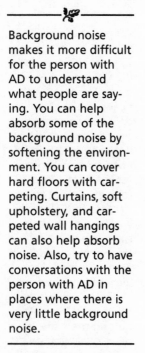

Background noise makes it more difficult for the person with AD to understand what people are saying. You can help absorb some of the background noise by softening the environment. You can cover hard floors with carpeting. Curtains, soft upholstery, and carpeted wall hangings can also help absorb noise. Also, try to have conversations with the person with AD in places where there is very little background noise.

Light sensors that turn on the light automatically as you approach a house are available to use outdoors and may help the person with AD when he or she leaves or returns home. These sensors may also be very useful in other parts of the house. They can be hooked up to closet doors, for example, so that when the person with AD opens the closet, the light will automatically turn on.

hot-water heater so that he cannot accidentally scald himself when turning on the water.

Radiators, floor heating vents, and other heating devices can also be very hot to the touch and therefore dangerous to the person with AD. Place protective radiator covers on radiators to prevent burns, or try to block access to radiators by placing a chair or another piece of furniture in front of them. Red tape around floor vents may deter the AD patient from standing on or touching the grid. Or, place a gate around a floor furnace or vent. It's best to not use space heaters, which can be easily touched or knocked over.

Incandescent light bulbs can also get very hot. In lamps that might get knocked over or touched by the person with AD, replace the incandescent bulbs with compact fluorescent bulbs that burn cooler. Also, halogen lamps are particularly dangerous because they burn very hot. Replace halogen lamps with lamps that use safer compact fluorescent bulbs.

## Is It Hazardous?

Many things around the house could be hazardous to the person with AD. Just as parents have to keep poisonous or hazardous materials away from small children, AD caregivers have to make sure that the person with AD does not have access to household items that might be dangerous. These include the following:

- Poisonous plants, such as philodendron and poinsettia (Check with local nurseries or poison centers for a list of poisonous plants.)
- Plastic bags with which the AD patient might choke or suffocate
- All guns, sharp knives, or other weapons
- Power tools and machinery
- Garden tools and garden chemicals
- All cleaning products
- All drugs and medications
- All flammable and volatile compounds

- Fish tanks
- All laundry products

If the person with AD smokes cigarettes, try not to let her continue to smoke. If you do let her smoke, make sure you monitor her when she is smoking. If you remove matches, cigarettes, and ashtrays from sight, the AD patient may forget her desire to smoke.

## Is It Sharp, Slippery, or in the Way?

Certain kinds of furniture and ordinary household objects may be more dangerous than others. In general, you should examine all furniture for sharp edges. Square or rectangular glass coffee tables and end tables can be particularly dangerous to the person with AD. Breakable items, such as lamps and framed pictures on tables, also might be dangerous. Other sharp objects that might be around the house include small objects, such as scissors, pins, needles, pencils, and letter openers.

You should also avoid using folding tables and chairs, which the affected person can trip over or knock over. All furniture should be arranged so that there are wide and easy pathways to navigate. And all hallways should be kept clear of furniture and other objects and clutter.

As the person with AD has more trouble with his or her coordination, you will need to make sure that the floors are not slippery. Don't polish or wax the floors. On hardwood floors, you can place textured strips or use nonskid wax to prevent falls. All small rugs and throw rugs in the house should also be removed, secured with nonskid backing, or tacked to the floor. Repair or replace any torn carpet and tack down the edges of the carpet.

Avoid the use of extension cords if possible by placing lamps and appliances close to electrical outlets. If you must use an extension cord, tack it to the baseboard so the AD patient won't trip on it. Unused outlets should be covered with childproof plugs. Don't use long telephone cords—if you don't already have a cordless phone, get one.

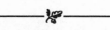

Many ordinary household items, if eaten or swallowed, can cause discomfort, illness, or even death. People with AD may not remember or understand that certain things—such as plants, cleaning products, soaps, spices, toothpaste, medications, alcoholic beverages, or other substances—should not be eaten or drunk, or at least not in large amounts. Make sure that you keep these potentially poisonous items in locked cabinets.

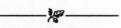

As a person with AD begins to develop visual difficulties, glass doors and windows can be very confusing. The Alzheimer's patient could inadvertently walk into or put a hand or foot through the glass. If you have sliding glass doors, storm doors, picture windows, or furniture with large glass panels, place decals on them at the AD patient's eye level to help him or her identify the glass pane.

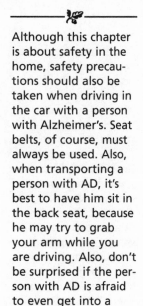

Although this chapter is about safety in the home, safety precautions should also be taken when driving in the car with a person with Alzheimer's. Seat belts, of course, must always be used. Also, when transporting a person with AD, it's best to have him sit in the back seat, because he may try to grab your arm while you are driving. Also, don't be surprised if the person with AD is afraid to even get into a vehicle.

## What Should Be Locked?

All hazardous materials should be locked away. That includes all medications, guns, knives, sharp objects, toxic chemicals such as cleaning products, and items the person can no longer use safely such as sewing machines, power tools, knives, shears, an iron, or a hair dryer. Alcohol should also be locked away because drinking it can lead to increased confusion.

In addition to locking away dangerous items, locks should be placed on your main fuse box and on controls for the thermostat and hot-water heater. Security locks should also be installed on windows and balcony doors. For your own convenience, you may want to lock the refrigerator so your loved one doesn't overeat or create a mess in the kitchen. You should also keep the door to the laundry room locked if possible. If not, keep all laundry products in a locked cabinet and then remove the knobs from the washer and dryer so the person with AD can't tamper with the machines. Keep the doors and lids to the washer and dryer closed and latched to prevent objects from being placed in the machines.

Remove all locks from inside rooms so that the affected person can't lock herself in or deny you access. It also might be a good idea to put electronic buzzers on doors so you know when the doors have been opened. Or, hang bells or chimes on doors leading to the outside so that you will know when the person with AD has gone out to wander.

You might also decide to lock the doors to the outside to prevent the person with AD from leaving the house and wandering the neighborhood. This might be very upsetting to the affected person, who has always been able to come and go as she pleased. In the interest of safety, however, it is probably better to keep the doors locked.

Car doors should be locked when you are not in the car. When you are in the car, if your car has a childproof locking system that prevents the person in the back seat from unlocking doors manually, that's great. If not, place heavy tape over knobs and handles to discourage the person with AD from attempting to open the door while you are driving. Keep all keys, and particularly your car keys, in a safe, locked area.

Remote controls will also disappear if you don't hide them or lock them away.

## Stairways

As a person with AD begins to have trouble with coordination, vision, and depth perception, stairs may become difficult for him or her to navigate without the possibility of accidents. To prevent the Alzheimer's patient from going up and down stairs you can install secure gates at both the top and the bottom of staircases. Of course, it makes sense to install gates across stairways only if you are sure the person will be unable to climb over them or open them without help.

In addition to installing gates, there are other measures you can take to keep the person with AD as safe as possible on stairways. First, remove any distractions—such as paintings, photographs, potted plants, floor decorations, or even wallpapers with interesting figures—on the stairs or stair walls. Second, add color to the forward edge of each step so there is a contrast to help the person with AD distinguish between the risers and the treads. This can be accomplished with safety grip strips, paint, or tape.

Also, make sure the steps are in good repair and that the railings are secure. Ideally, there should be railings that are easy to grip on both sides of stairways, and the railings should extend beyond the first and last steps. If the steps have carpeting on them, make sure that it isn't worn or loose. Finally, light switches should be placed at the top and bottom of staircases.

## The Bathroom

Bathrooms can be particularly dangerous places for people with Alzheimer's. In the later stages of the disease, it's better to not even let the person with AD go into the bathroom alone. Locks should be removed from the door to prevent the affected person from getting locked in the room. Medication should be stored in a locked cabinet or drawer and any cleaning products should be removed from under the sink or locked in a cabinet.

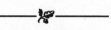

There are tricks to installing locks that you might want to consider. Locate locks in places where the person with AD is less likely to notice them, such as in the upper or lower corners of doors. Also, try putting more than one lock on the door, making the process of opening the door more time-consuming and confusing for the AD patient. Opening the door might take long enough for you to discover he or she is about to go wandering. You can also use different types of locks that require different skills to open, which may be too complicated for your loved one to figure out. Your local locksmith may be able to make some recommendations about hard-to-lock doors and windows and may also be the perfect person to install these devices for you.

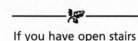

If you have open stairs in your home—which are stairs that have no risers or vertical parts, only horizontal treads—they can be particularly difficult for people with AD. Distractions can be seen through the steps that might confuse the affected person. These types of stairs can also trigger a fear of heights. If they can't be closed by adding plates to the back of each stair, then they should be gated.

All small electrical appliances should be removed from the bathroom and electrical outlets should be covered. If a male patient uses an electric shaver, have him use a mirror outside the bathroom to avoid water contact or make sure the razor is waterproof. Mirrors themselves are sometimes frightening to people with Alzheimer's, and you may have to cover them.

In addition to these precautions, certain kinds of equipment and devices should be installed in the bathroom to make it safer. These include …

- Handrails and grab bars in and around the tub—in colors that contrast with the wall.
- A bath bench, plastic seat, or chair for the shower or tub.
- A hand-held showerhead to make bathing easier.
- Nonskid adhesive strips, decals, or mats on the tub floor to prevent slipping.
- Nonskid adhesive strips next to the tub, toilet, and sink.
- Washable wall-to-wall bathroom carpeting to prevent slipping.
- An extended toilet seat with handrails, or grab rails at the side of the toilet.
- Light switches that can be easily reached, and a night-light.
- A shower curtain to replace glass shower doors.
- A foam rubber faucet cover in the tub to prevent injury should the AD patient fall.
- Drain traps in sinks to catch small items that may be lost.
- A single faucet that mixes hot and cold water in the shower, tub, and sink to avoid scalding.
- An intercom device similar to those used in babies' rooms, so you can hear if the person needs help.
- Covers for mirrors—although you may remove the mirrors instead.

When the person with AD uses a wheelchair, these additional changes should be made:

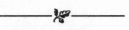

- Install wheelchair-accessible sinks and mirrors if possible. The sink should be 24 inches from the floor.
- Insulate exposed hot-water pipes under the sink to protect the person's legs.
- If you do not already have toilet guardrails or an elevated toilet seat, you will need them, since most toilet seats are too low for people who use wheelchairs.
- Place a regular chair under the sink if there isn't enough room for a wheelchair.

## The Bedroom

Certain safety precautions should also be taken in the affected person's bedroom. If the Alzheimer's patient's bedroom is on the second floor of the house, think about moving him to the first floor so he doesn't have to go up or down the stairs frequently.

As in other rooms, make sure there are no sharp objects, that the floors are not slippery, and that you have removed or tacked down any small rugs. Also, make sure the room is generally well-lighted and that a night-light is on at night.

Since falling out of bed is a common problem with AD patients, you can reduce the risk by placing the bed against the wall. Also put a mattress or futon next to the bed on the floor to reduce the impact if the affected person does fall. Unless the person with AD is completely bedridden, a hospital bed with railings is not recommended because the individual might try to climb out of it and fall. If you do use a hospital bed, make sure the brakes are locked.

You should also be very cautious about using electric mattress pads, electric blankets, or heating pads, all of which may cause burns. If you must use them, keep the controls out of the AD patient's reach. Portable space heaters should not be used in a room where the patient sleeps alone. Also, portable fans are not safe for AD patients.

As in the bathroom, you might want to install an intercom device to alert you to any noises that might indicate the need

As AD progresses, a person with the disease will develop problems with balance or muscle weakness. It's very important, therefore, to put a bench or plastic seat in the shower or tub. The seat should be the same height as a wheelchair, approximately 19 inches. Some tub seats have adjustable legs or back supports. If you can't get a tub seat, place a sturdy chair with rubber tips on the legs in the tub or shower stall.

────────── ❧ ──────────

When the person with AD uses a wheelchair and is still able to dress himself, his closet—if it is accessible to a wheelchair—should be adjusted so that he has easy access to his clothes. Clothing should be hung on lower rods that are no more than 36 inches from the floor. Shoes and accessories can be placed in shoe bags that hang from the door or the lower rod.

for help. A telephone or emergency buzzer should also be within easy reach of the bed.

## The Kitchen

The kitchen can, of course, also be a particularly dangerous place for a person with Alzheimer's disease. Here are some guidelines for keeping the kitchen safe:

- Don't wax the kitchen floor.
- Remove any scatter rugs or foam pads from the floor.
- To prevent burns, use pots and pans with handles that don't conduct heat.
- Install childproof safety latches and locks on all cabinets and drawers with breakable or dangerous items.
- Remove knobs from the stove or install an automatic shut-off switch.
- Because they are safer than conventional range ovens, use a microwave or toaster oven for cooking when possible.
- Eliminate inedible items that look like food, such as artificial fruits and vegetables or food-shaped kitchen magnets.
- Install tamper-proof water faucets.
- Place a drain trap in the kitchen sink to catch anything that may clog the plumbing or become lost.
- Consider dismantling the garbage disposal, since AD patients may place objects or their hands into the disposal.
- Don't leave hot coffee pots on the counter. Use a thermos to keep coffee warm.
- Lock away all dangerous items—household cleaning products, matches, sharp knives, scissors, erasers, blades, toothpicks, plastic bags, spice bottles, small appliances, and valued china.

# Outdoors

You should also make sure that your yard and outdoor areas are not dangerous for the person with AD. At least a portion of the yard should be a safe area, so the person with AD can enjoy the outdoors. Fences should be high enough that the affected person cannot get over them, and gates should be locked and difficult for the person to open. Walkways should be safe and clear of toys, fallen branches, newspapers, or other clutter. You should check for uneven ground, cracked pavement, or other conditions that might cause the affected person to trip. Also, make sure your lawn furniture is sturdy.

If you have a patio area and grill, remove the fuel source and fire starters from the grill when not in use and be watchful when the AD patient is present. If there are steps to a porch or deck, paint them in bright, contrasting colors so that they are clearly visible. Install a banister if it seems necessary in order to prevent falls.

You might have to monitor the person with AD when she is outdoors. The affected person may eat flowers, weeds, or dirt or trip on uneven ground or stones. Also, let your neighbors and local authorities know that your loved one has Alzheimer's, so they can be on alert if she wanders.

# Other Issues

In addition to safeguarding the home, it's important to have an emergency plan ready in case something does happen. What will you do if the person falls and is hurt? Keep a list of emergency phone numbers next to each phone and make sure you have a complete first aid kit.

## Fire Safety

Fire safety is important in any home, but in the home of a person with AD, it is particularly important because of the

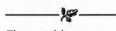

The outside approaches to the house should be safe for the person with AD. Make sure you keep stairs sturdy and textured to prevent falls in wet or icy weather. Also, use bright or reflective tape to mark the edges of stairs. A ramp with handrails into the home may be better than stairs. Consider a "No Solicitation" sign for the front door. Keep bushes and foliage pruned well away from the walkways and doorways.

chance that the confused person might set a fire. Here are some steps you can take to reduce the risk:

- Place smoke alarms throughout the house, including the basement and bedrooms.
- Place a fire extinguisher on each floor.
- Put safety caps over all electrical outlets.
- Keep all matches and lighters out of reach.
- Use flame-retardant sheets and mattresses.
- Check fire extinguishers and smoke alarm batteries monthly.
- Don't leave the person with AD alone near an open fireplace.

## Memory Aids

We have focused on safety issues in this chapter, but you also need to make changes to your home to help the person with AD remember where things are and where he or she is. Large, easy to read signs on drawers and doors may help the person with AD find belongings or not get lost.

Since the person with AD is also unlikely to remember messages, you should have some type of phone answering system when you are unable to answer calls. In addition to forgetting messages, the AD patient may be an easy target for exploitation by phone solicitors.

We have covered a lot of safety issues in this chapter. You may not feel that all of this information applies to your loved one, but as her behavior and abilities change, you may need to reevaluate your home safety precautions. The next chapter discusses another potentially difficult subject in caring for a person with AD at home—mealtimes.

# 18

# *Mealtime Traumas*

---

Why is the simple act of eating sometimes traumatic for the person with Alzheimer's disease? We often don't realize that there are a number of actions that a person must remember in order to eat in a civilized way, because eating is something we learned at a very young age. First, a person needs to feel hunger and remember that eating satisfies hunger. The person then needs to carry out a series of actions in order to eat—sit at a table, use certain utensils to put food onto his plate, use other utensils to move the food from the plate to his mouth, chew the food, swallow the food, and then use a utensil to get more food.

For those of us without the memory loss caused by AD, the steps in this process seem simple. For a person with AD, however, remembering all of those steps may be difficult. As the disease destroys brain cells and memory, any part of the process may be forgotten. He may forget that eating takes away hunger. He may not remember where to eat, how to use various utensils, or what to do once the food is in his mouth. In this chapter, you'll learn how you, as a caregiver, can help the person with AD have an easier time eating and minimize the traumas that might occur at mealtime.

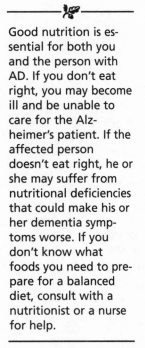

Good nutrition is essential for both you and the person with AD. If you don't eat right, you may become ill and be unable to care for the Alzheimer's patient. If the affected person doesn't eat right, he or she may suffer from nutritional deficiencies that could make his or her dementia symptoms worse. If you don't know what foods you need to prepare for a balanced diet, consult with a nutritionist or a nurse for help.

When shopping for the Alzheimer's patient, remember that certain foods with caffeine, such as coffee, cola products, and tea may interfere with sleep. Even alcohol, which may initially be relaxing, can cause patients to wake up in the night as the effect of the alcohol diminishes. Also, give the affected person water to quench her thirst before meals, because drinking juice, fruit punch, or soda can make her too full for a healthy meal or snack.

# Planning and Preparing Meals

Planning and preparing all meals is a difficult job, and it may be a job that you haven't done on a regular basis before. Nevertheless, as chief cook and caregiver, you must find ways to provide both you and the person with AD with good, balanced nutrition.

A meal with an Alzheimer's patient is more complicated than just cooking for someone who is ill. When you are taking care of a person with Alzheimer's disease, you might spend a lot of time and effort slaving over the stove to prepare a meal only to have him tell you that he is not hungry and doesn't want the food. If you persist, the affected person might throw your meal on the floor. So with Alzheimer's, your job is not only to plan and prepare all of the meals, it's also to figure out how to get the affected person to eat them. To do that, you must figure out what kind of food to serve and how to prepare it, as well as when and how to serve the meals.

## What to Serve

There is no special diet that will alleviate the symptoms of AD, but the affected person still needs a good, balanced diet to function as well as he or she can. Within the bounds of getting good nutrition, try to serve her favorite foods often, especially if she doesn't seem interested in food. Variety isn't as important as making sure the person with AD is getting enough calories and enough of the basic food groups.

If the person with AD didn't like a particular food before she was diagnosed, she probably won't like it afterward, either. Serving her familiar and favorite foods can help ease mealtime difficulties and ensure that she gets proper nutrition. Continue to pay attention to how she reacts to what you serve, however, because her food preferences may change during the progression of the disease. In addition to preparing food that the person with AD likes, make sure that you cook the food the way she likes it—even though it may not be the way you like it.

If the food the affected person wants isn't particularly nutritious or if she only eats a little food, you can always spike it with extra nutrients. For example, wheat germ can be added to soups, shredded carrots and celery to tuna fish, cheese to salads, and protein powder to milk shakes. Nutritional supplements and vitamins also provide extra nutrients. Ask the doctor for a list of supplements that are best for your loved one. If the affected person is not eating enough nutritious food, you might also want to add to her diet a nutritional supplement like Ensure, Ensure Plus, or Meritene. You can doctor it with some frozen yogurt or ice cream and not even tell her that she is getting a nutritional supplement.

Make sure that the meals you prepare include a protein source (meat, fish, chicken, or beans), a dairy product (milk, yogurt, or cheese), a starch (rice, potato, peas, corn, or bread), vegetables, and fruit. If you provide enough variety, the affected person will get plenty of nutrients, no matter how much he or she chooses to eat.

People with Alzheimer's disease often like sweet foods and fruit. Keep a bowl of fruit available for snacks throughout the day and serve fruit as dessert. Finger foods, such as raw fruits and vegetables cut into slices, are also good because the person with AD does not have to struggle with utensils. Sandwiches cut up into quarters are also easy meals for the affected person to eat.

## When to Eat

The important thing about meals, as with other activities in an Alzheimer's patient's life, is that they be on a regular schedule. A set routine each day will be easier for the person with AD to handle than spontaneous or changing mealtimes.

Also, small meals at regular intervals throughout the day may be better for a person with AD than three large ones. It is often difficult for Alzheimer's patients—or anyone—to digest large amounts of food, so a number of smaller, nutritious meals or snacks are good. Some ideas for healthy snacks include fruits, peanut butter, applesauce, yogurt, tuna, and cheese and crackers.

Even if you regularly prepare meals, with the additional responsibilities of caring for the Alzheimer's patient, you may not feel like cooking every night. Give yourself regular time off. See if you qualify for the Meals-on-Wheels program in your area. If not, find a restaurant you like and get takeout food. When you do cook, make large amounts and freeze portions for later. It's best to avoid frozen dinners unless you know that the particular brand provides well-balanced meals.

———————🦋———————

Although most experts recommend serving each food item separately, some caregivers have had success putting small portions of all the food, including dessert, on the plate at the beginning of the meal and letting the affected person eat in whatever order he or she wishes. Some people will eat more if the food is served in this way—even if the dessert is eaten first. You may have to experiment a bit to see what works for your loved one.

## At the Table

There are things you can do to help the person with AD feel more comfortable when he sits down at the table to eat. People with Alzheimer's disease will begin to have difficulty with coordination and vision. To help the affected person distinguish everything on the table, make sure that the dishes, the tablecloth, and the place mats differ in color from the food. The idea is to make the food, dishes, and table surface all look different from each other. Use plain dishes with no design or pattern.

Eating with one or two other people at a small table in a quiet room is ideal for the person with AD. It is depressing to eat alone, and to eat with a large number of people—as at a restaurant—is usually too distracting. Make sure that each person has the same place at the table each night.

With the loss of memory and coordination that the Alzheimer's patient suffers from, spills and messes are inevitable, so meals should be served in an area that is easy to clean. If the floor under the table is not easy to clean, you can place a tarp or large plastic tablecloth on the floor. With the person's permission, you can have him wear a large apron or a smock during the meal. Or, he can wear clothes that are easy to clean or already stained.

Keep the food you prepare simple—too many choices can be confusing for the person with AD. Among the foods that you do prepare for a meal, offer one item at a time to the person with AD and let him choose how much of each food he wants.

Some other tips for making mealtimes easier for the person with AD include ...

- Provide enough light to see the food—but not bright, glaring light.
- Make sure there are no unpleasant smells at mealtime, such as the odor of cleaning products.
- Make sure the food looks good and smells good.
- Try placing nonskid material under plates and bowls to make eating as easy as possible.
- Use unbreakable plastic dishes.

- If the person often knocks dishes off the table, try using plates and cups with suction cups on them (available at baby stores).
- Remove other distracting items from the table, including salt and pepper shakers or other condiment holders.
- Use only one utensil, either a fork or a spoon, for the duration of the meal.
- Before serving them, cut certain foods, such as meat, into bite-sized pieces.
- Don't give the person a lot of food at one time.
- Serve soup in a cup—it's easier than handling a bowl and a spoon.
- Don't insist that the person with AD eat if he or she is tired or irritable.
- Allow individuals to feed themselves as much as possible.

## How to Eat

The person with AD may forget many actions that are part of how we eat—how to sit in a chair at the table, how to use utensils, how to chew, and how to swallow. You may have to show him how to eat again at each meal—and even over again in the middle of a meal.

The first step in showing the affected person how to eat is to make sure that he is seated comfortably at the table—or in an easy chair or bed if the person cannot eat at the table. Once seated comfortably, if a person is not eating, try modeling eating behavior. First, get his attention; then take a piece of food from your plate and put it in your mouth while looking at him. Then, ask him to do what you are doing.

If the person with AD can eat on his own, you should know which utensils are easiest for him to use. You may have to cut his food into small pieces. It's best to do that in the kitchen to prevent possible embarrassment. Also, people with AD often lose the ability to judge the temperature of food; so before you serve the person with AD, make sure that you check it to see whether it's too hot or too cold.

Sometimes an Alzheimer's patient will hoard food, hiding it in her room or some other hiding place. The person may feel anxious that the food won't be available when she wants it. This is a problem because the forgotten food can attract insects or mice. To help prevent hoarding, reassure the person that she can have a snack at any time, keep a container filled with snack foods out in easy view and remind her where it is frequently.

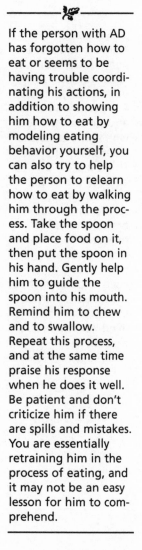

If the person with AD has forgotten how to eat or seems to be having trouble coordinating his actions, in addition to showing him how to eat by modeling eating behavior yourself, you can also try to help the person to relearn how to eat by walking him through the process. Take the spoon and place food on it, then put the spoon in his hand. Gently help him to guide the spoon into his mouth. Remind him to chew and to swallow. Repeat this process, and at the same time praise his response when he does it well. Be patient and don't criticize him if there are spills and mistakes. You are essentially retraining him in the process of eating, and it may not be an easy lesson for him to comprehend.

# Other Mealtime Problems

As the person with AD advances into the middle and late stages of the disease, he might begin to hoard food or eat non-food items, such as soap or plants. The affected person may also become very finicky about what he will eat and may find new foods confusing.

The Alzheimer's patient may also have physical conditions that affect his or her ability to eat. One example is some type of mouth discomfort, such as sore teeth, loose dentures, or dryness of the mouth. Or, the affected person may be taking medications that are causing certain side effects that affect his or her appetite or ability to eat. He or she may be constipated, depressed or agitated or may be suffering from a chronic or acute illness. And, of course, the memory loss from Alzheimer's disease itself may cause the person to be unable to recognize the sensation of hunger. She may also forget how to eat with utensils or forget that she has eaten right after a meal.

If a person with AD has difficulties at meals, try to look for patterns. Does she have particular difficulties with certain foods? Does she have chewing or swallowing problems? Does she seem more agitated around certain people? You will be able to make changes that can alleviate the problem when you know its source.

*One Caregiver's Journey*

"When my mother lived at the senior residence, she took all of her meals in the dining room. She was very good about that, but she didn't seem to be comfortable eating anywhere else. When she came to my house, she seemed to know that she was at my house, but she always wanted to go home shortly after she got here. One Thanksgiving, we had barely sat down for dinner and she said, 'I want to go home.' I said, 'Well, we haven't had our dinner yet. Wait until after dinner.' She said, 'No, I want to go home now.' So I left everyone to eat and drove her home."

# Choking

As the disease progresses, the person with AD may develop difficulty chewing and swallowing, so it's important to serve foods that don't need much chewing and are as easy to swallow as possible. These include soups, bananas, cottage cheese, scrambled eggs, ground meat, mashed potatoes, applesauce, and pureed vegetables. Solid foods alone are also better than combined foods, such as cereal and milk. Never serve tough meat or crunchy snacks like hard candy or nuts. You may have to learn how to use a food processor and develop some new recipes to accommodate this difficulty.

Some caregivers use baby foods as substitutes for meat, vegetables, and fruits that are hard to chew. Baby foods are expensive and may be both uninteresting and insulting to the person with AD, so be careful. If you must use baby foods, supplement them with dairy products, such as cottage cheese and yogurt.

When the person with AD has developed problems with chewing and swallowing, you have to be ready for the possibility of choking. No matter what kind of soft and easy-to-swallow foods you serve to try to prevent choking, it might happen anyway. Be prepared by learning the Heimlich maneuver, which is a technique to clear the air passages of a choking person. Your doctor or the local Red Cross may know of classes that can teach you the technique.

The risk of choking increases later in the day when the person with AD is tired, so be especially careful of foods served at dinner and in the evening. If the person starts to choke, don't slap his back because it may actually cause the food in the throat to be lodged there more permanently instead of dislodging it.

## Feeding Someone Who Is Bedridden

If the person with AD is not able to get out of bed but still lives at home, there are several things you should do at mealtime. The following tips might help:

Most people with Alzheimer's take various kinds of medications, and some AD patients may forget how to swallow pills. Others may spit them out, give them to the dog, or hide them. To insure that the affected person takes his or her medication, crush the pill and put it in applesauce, scrambled eggs, oatmeal, or any food with both a strong enough flavor to hide the taste and a consistency that is easy to swallow.

———— ❧ ————

Learn the Heimlich maneuver from a professional, but if you haven't yet and an emergency occurs, here are the basic steps:

1. Step behind the person and clasp your hands around his abdomen below the rib cage. Make sure your hands are in the soft abdomen below the rib cage.

2. Make a fist with one hand and hold the thumb side against the person's abdomen.

3. Grasp the fist with your other hand and thrust it forcefully in and up.

4. If one forceful thrust doesn't dislodge the piece of food and restore breathing, repeat the procedure.

5. If this doesn't work, lay the person down face-up and apply upper abdominal thrusts with the heel of your hand, then turn the person's head sideways and check the mouth for food.

6. If there is still a problem, call 911. The operator will send help and talk you through CPR.

- Elevate the person's head with pillows, and always support the person's head because eating while lying down can lead to choking.
- Use a bendable straw or drinking tube for liquids.
- Serve lukewarm foods that need very little chewing.
- Feed him or her with a half-full spoon and wait at least five seconds before offering more food.
- Protect sheets with a plastic cover, such as a plastic bag, placed under the food tray.
- The person should be kept sitting upright for at least a half-hour after eating to avoid choking on food if she falls asleep.

# Drinking

Even people in the early stages of AD forget to drink enough fluids and can become dehydrated. See Chapter 14, "Medical Care Issues in Stage 3," for a list of the symptoms of dehydration. It's important that you pay attention to the amount of fluids that the person with AD drinks.

If she doesn't like water, offer juice and remind her to take more than just a few sips. Avoid caffeinated drinks, because they are diuretics—they take fluids from the body. Some medications, such as those taken for the heart or for diabetes, are also diuretics. If the affected person is taking a diuretic, she must drink even more fluids.

# 19

# *Personal Hygiene at Home*

As Alzheimer's disease progresses into the middle and late stages, your loved one will begin to lose the ability to take care of himself in the most basic, personal ways. This is, of course, very upsetting for both you the caregiver and the person with AD, because personal hygiene is just that—it's personal. It's something we normally do for ourselves in the privacy of our own bathroom and bedroom.

Although the amount of personal care an AD patient will need varies with the individual, most people with the disease will eventually depend on the caregiver for some type of help with all of the basic, personal, daily routines—from getting dressed to using the toilet. The resulting lack of privacy is something both you and the person with AD will have to find ways to adjust to.

How can you best help your loved one with Alzheimer's in these personal matters? The following sections present some ideas that other caregivers have found helpful. In addition to reading this chapter, you also can ask an occupational thera-pist or home-care nurse for tips on how to perform personal care tasks safely and effectively.

*One Caregiver's Journey*

"A person in my support group told a story about a man who had been an actor all of his life and who now had Alzheimer's disease. His daughter was taking care of him and when he began to resist bathing and dressing, she was very upset. She talked to a nurse who suggested that she use his former career to get him to cooperate in getting dressed and bathed. So, every morning, his daughter would tell him that his agent had called to say he had an audition scheduled for later that afternoon. She then asked him if he wanted to get bathed and dressed so he would be ready for the audition. He immediately agreed and without any protest took his bath and allowed his daughter to help him dress. He was clean and spiffy every day. By the time the afternoon rolled around, however, he had forgotten all about the audition."

# Getting Dressed

Physical appearance is important to all of us. It bolsters self-esteem when we look good, and it can make us feel depressed when we don't. For the person with Alzheimer's, however, the act of getting dressed can be very frustrating. As you learned in earlier chapters, there are many reasons why the person with AD might have problems dressing. They include physical problems, such as those caused by the loss of motor skills; memory problems, such as not remembering how to dress; environmental problems, such as a lack of privacy, a cold room, poor lighting, or loud noises; or other issues, such as the pressure to dress quickly.

## How You Can Help

Chapter 7, "What to Expect in Stage 1," explains the signs that clue you in to the fact that the person with AD is having trouble dressing. He might start wearing unmatched clothing, or might wear his clothing backward or wear dirty clothes.

How do you help? Some of the following suggestions might help you assist the person with AD:

- Allow the person to be as independent as possible, even if dressing takes more time than it would with your help.
- If the person needs help getting dressed, give step-by-step instructions and take one step at a time.
- Try arranging clothes by laying them out on the bed in the order they are to be put on.
- Encourage the person to choose his or her own clothes, but make the choice easier by organizing the closet and limiting the choices.
- Maintain a routine for getting dressed that is followed every day.
- Choose one spot to dress and another spot to undress, and keep them consistent.
- Make sure the bedroom or dressing area is free of clutter.
- Be sensitive to the temperature of the room—if it's too warm the person may take clothing off, and if it's too cool he may not want to undress. Also, even though you may feel that it is oppressively hot inside the house, the Alzheimer's patient might find the temperature comfortable.
- Keep the room well-lighted while the person dresses.
- Insure privacy as much as possible—close curtains and doors and don't be there unless you have to.
- Be flexible and ready to try new approaches, providing additional assistance as the person becomes more impaired.
- Don't argue or try to force a person to change clothes.
- Don't rush the person while he or she is dressing.

Being reminded to change clothes can be humiliating and might upset the person with AD, so do it as gently as possible. Also, remember that in the past many people didn't change clothes as often as we do today, and we shouldn't necessarily impose our values on older people.

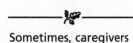

Sometimes, caregivers combine several small steps together, not realizing that the affected person may no longer be able to do two or three steps at once. For example, you might hand the person pants to put on, not realizing that he first has to distinguish the front from the back, then put a leg into each pant leg, and finally pull them up to his waist. You may have to gently remind him of each step in the process.

Whenever possible, include the Alzheimer's patient in making plans for her care. Take her suggestions and feelings into consideration, and encourage her involvement. If she can't perform a certain activity, see if there is part of it that she can do by herself. For example, she might be able to independently dress her upper body if sitting, but may require your help dressing her lower body.

## What to Wear

Although Chapter 7 covers some suggestions for the kinds of clothes the person with AD should wear, we'll go over those ideas, as well as other suggestions, here. In general, clothing for the person with AD should be comfortable, attractive, and easy to put on and remove.

The following suggestions will help you put together a wardrobe for the person with AD that is easier to handle and safer to wear:

- Jogging suits or sweat pants in attractive colors are easy to get into and out of, and are comfortable.
- Shoes with nonskid soles that either slip on or have Velcro closures. (Tennis shoes with Velcro closures work well.)
- Pants or skirts with elastic waistbands.
- Over-the-head, loose-fitting clothing.
- Soft and loosely constructed underwear.
- Tube socks, rather than tight socks that can cut off circulation.
- Clothing in solid, contrasting colors, rather than busy designs or patterns.
- Clothing that is washable and doesn't need ironing.
- Clothing with Velcro tape in place of buttons, snaps, hooks, zippers, and belt buckles, which are hard to manipulate.
- Clothing that fits comfortably—in larger or looser styles, rather than tightly fitting styles or sizes.
- Clothes that are not too long, to avoid tripping and falling.

- Clothing that is up-to-date, clean, color-coordinated, and neat.
- Clothing in comfortable fabrics like cotton, rather than wool and other fabrics that can feel scratchy. As clothes wear out, replace them with machine washable, non-restrictive, no-iron items.
- Watch for changing size needs as the person gains or loses weight.
- T-shirts for casual wear—they look okay even if worn backward.

For women with Alzheimer's disease, there are some special considerations. A bra might be difficult for a woman with AD to put on by herself. Consider whether or not it is really necessary. Could you substitute a cotton vest, an undershirt, or a T-shirt? Remember, however, that she may have worn a bra all of her life and might feel embarrassed or uncomfortable about being without one.

Rather than panty hose, which can be difficult to put on, or knee-highs with wide elastic bands, which may be bad for people with circulation problems, try short cotton socks, or knee-high or thigh-high stockings. Don't bother with a slip unless the affected person feels uncomfortable without it. For a woman who is used to wearing jewelry each day, a simple necklace with no clasps might help preserve her self-esteem.

Some AD patients will want to wear the same outfit day after day. If so, don't argue, but instead buy similar outfits and substitute them when the first one is dirty.

Dressing may be somewhat easier for the person with AD if his or her closet is well-organized. Here are some tips for organizing the closet. Clothing should be stored so it is easy to reach. Sort and arrange all clothing by type—hang all skirts together, all pants together, and all shirts together. Hangers that serve the same purpose should have the same design. All pants or skirt hangers, for example, should have either clips or pressure bars. Put ties, scarves, belts or sashes, and other accessories with the item of clothing they go with. If you find that a particular item causes confusion, adapt it or get rid of it.

—————— ✤ ——————

Grooming, like bathing and dressing a person with AD, takes a lot of patience. You may feel tempted to skip some aspect of the regular routine because it's just too frustrating. It's better, however, to keep the affected person as presentable as possible. It helps the AD patient feel better about herself and may improve her mood and her cooperation with you. It also might help if you compliment her on her appearance from time to time.

For example, if a woman forgets how to tie a scarf, either fasten it to her dress already tied or remove it altogether. In the drawer, keep all socks together, all underpants together, and all nightwear together, and label the drawer.

## Still Having Problems?

If you have tried everything and the person with AD still has difficulty dressing, he or she may have medical or physical problems that are contributing to the problems dressing, such as reactions to medications. Have the person get a medical checkup to discover any possible causes. The person may have impaired vision, so have vision or glasses checked. Also, have the person evaluated for depression, particularly if he or she is frequently unwilling to get up or get dressed in the morning.

# Personal Grooming

Our grooming contributes to how we look and feel about ourselves. Therefore, it's important that the Alzheimer's patient's personal grooming not be neglected. As with dressing, no matter how small the activity—holding the soap, combing the front of his or her hair—it's important that the person be able to participate and do as much as she can independently.

## Hair

Keep the person's hair cut in an easy-to-care-for style. If the barbershop or beauty parlor has been an important part of the person's former routine, continue to let her go to the same place, at a regular appointment time, for as long as possible. As for washing her hair, that may be easier to do at the kitchen sink than in the tub or shower. A hose or spray attachment can be put on the faucet to make rinsing easier.

## Shaving and Make-Up

It may be difficult to shave the person yourself, so try to get him to shave as long as possible, with you supervising the activity. Getting him to use an electric razor may simplify the process. For a woman with AD, in addition to helping her shave her legs and underarms, you may need to help her pluck or shave her chin if she has facial hair.

Most women stop using make-up early in the disease, but a woman who has worn make-up every day will feel better about herself if she continues using it. Use a little lipstick and a bit of powder, but forget the eye make-up—it's too hard to put on.

## Nails

Encourage the person with Alzheimer's to continue trimming his or her fingernails and toenails. When you must take over, do it a couple of times a month. You may get more cooperation if you trim his or her nails while the person is listening to music or otherwise distracted. If the person has difficulty with toenails, bunions, or calluses, it might cause not only discomfort, but also problems with walking. In those cases, a regular visit to a podiatrist is a good idea.

## Oral Hygiene

Make sure the person brushes his or her teeth at least twice a day. You may have to help, but let the person do as much of the task as possible. If you have to take over brushing his or her teeth, consult with your dentist as to how to best do it. If he or she has dentures, they must be cleaned daily and they must adhere properly. Ill-fitting dentures can contribute to poor nutrition and result in constipation or mouth sores. Continue to schedule regular visits to the dentist as long as possible.

# Bathing

While some people with Alzheimer's disease enjoy the soothing relaxation of being in the bathtub, bathing can be frightening, complicated, and overwhelming for many other people in the middle and late stages of the disease. Helping the person with AD take a bath or a shower can often be a challenging task for the caregiver. How can bathing be accomplished with the greatest success for both the person with the disease and for you?

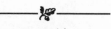

For success with bathing, it helps to know the person's prior bathing routine. The more familiar and comfortable he or she is, the greater the likelihood of success. Some questions to consider are: Did he or she usually take a shower or a bath? In the morning or evening? Was he or she always very private or modest? Would the person feel more comfortable and safe with a same-sex caregiver?

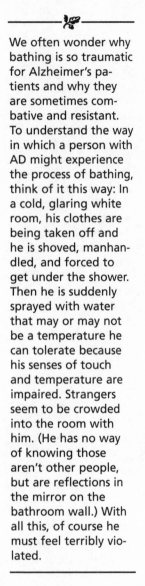

We often wonder why bathing is so traumatic for Alzheimer's patients and why they are sometimes combative and resistant. To understand the way in which a person with AD might experience the process of bathing, think of it this way: In a cold, glaring white room, his clothes are being taken off and he is shoved, manhandled, and forced to get under the shower. Then he is suddenly sprayed with water that may or may not be a temperature he can tolerate because his senses of touch and temperature are impaired. Strangers seem to be crowded into the room with him. (He has no way of knowing those aren't other people, but are reflections in the mirror on the bathroom wall.) With all this, of course he must feel terribly violated.

First, you need to know the reasons bathing can be so stressful for a person with AD. Bathing, like eating, is a complicated task with many steps, and when confronted with it, the affected person may feel overwhelmed. Or, the person may think he or she has already taken a shower and so now doesn't need one. The AD patient may be upset by the bathroom environment—the glare of the lights, the cold white tile floors, white tub, white shower stall, the confusing mirrors, or the loud sound of the water running and people talking over it.

As the disease progresses, people with Alzheimer's lose depth perception and may not realize that the water in the tub is only four inches deep. The affected person may fear drowning and refuse to get into the tub. Other fears may be present, such as fear of the sound of running water or of the water itself, fear of soap, or fear of shampoo.

If the person is modest or shy, he or she may feel upset about the lack of privacy and may resist if you try to take his or her clothes off. The person with AD may misunderstand the purpose of bathing. Or, he or she may deny needing any help. And if you try to force him or her to see things your way, it only causes further confusion and agitation. Depression also can cause a lack of interest in bathing and other aspects of personal care.

## Preparing the Bath

Before you start to give the affected person a bath, make sure the bathroom is a safe and inviting environment. (See Chapter 17, "Securing Your Home," for modifications that should be made to the bathroom.) Be sure that the room is warm, but not hot and humid. Be sure that the light in the room is bright, but not glaring. Be sure that the room isn't cluttered. Don't leave hair dryers, razors, or glass bottles within reach of the person with AD.

Many people prefer a shower to a bath—it's easier and feels safer, but the best thing for your loved one is whatever he or she is used to. If you use a tub, fill it with four to six inches of water and stay with the person while he or she is bathing.

Don't use slippery oils or bubble bath. If the person is agitated when he enters the tub because he hasn't seen it being filled, then let him stay in the room while the water fills the tub. If running water frightens him, fill the tub with four inches of water, and when it's filled, lead him to the bathroom and into the tub.

Make sure everything is ready ahead of time—bath water, towels, clothes—before you bring the person with AD into the bathroom. Also, keep things quiet when you take him or her into the bathroom. Speak in calm, loving, supportive tones, and keep good eye contact with him or her.

## Tips for Successful Bathing

Here are some strategies for dealing with bathing that other caregivers have found successful:

- Pick a day and time when the person is in a good mood and not upset or frustrated.

- Approach him or her in a calm, gentle, and nonthreatening manner. Begin a conversation, but don't focus on the bath right away.

- Plan the bath when you are not feeling rushed. If he or she is uncooperative, try again later.

- Consider giving the person a reason for the bath that makes sense to him or her. For instance, say, "It's time to get ready for work."

- Schedule the bath at a time when the person is already engaged in a related activity, such as in the morning before getting dressed or at night when getting undressed.

- Make sure you have everything you need in advance so you don't have to leave the bathroom after you start the bath.

- Go slowly and say out loud each step you are taking in simple terms.

- Focus on the person's mood and behavior, rather than on the task itself.

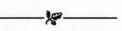

When an Alzheimer's patient resists getting undressed, encourage him by talking about what is to come as a reward—a nice refreshing bath or a cool, comfortable bed. Or, try to distract him with a funny story or song. When he clutches his clothing so it can't be removed, put something in his hands like a glass of milk or a book to draw his attention away. As soon as the clothes are off, take them out of his view.

—— ❧ ——

Bathing a relative with AD can be challenging because of the role change it represents. For example, bathing one's mother or husband isn't part of the usual relationship. If you are anxious or embarrassed, it may cause the AD patient to also feel anxious. Consider hiring someone to help if the act of bathing is too physically or emotionally overwhelming for you to do alone. Or, enlist the help of another family member who is more comfortable with the task.

- Encourage the person to help as much as possible and give him or her something to hold on to, such as a washcloth, towel, or grab bar, to lessen the feeling of being out of control.
- Praise the person and let him or her know that the task is going well.
- If the person is modest, try keeping him or her partially covered with a towel or shower blanket.
- If the person has depth perception problems, keep the tub drained of water and use a flexible shower hose.
- Wash the person's body in the same order every time.

## Dealing with Problems

What do you do when the person with AD becomes frightened or threatened before or during bathing? If the person begins hitting or striking out, it may be that he or she feels frightened and needs to defend himself or herself. Try to prevent this agitation from escalating. If you can, find out the cause of the person's anxiety and remove it. If you can't figure out what is causing the problem, try to distract the person. Also, keep reassuring the affected person—telling her she is safe. It may take two people to help with the AD patient's bath—one to focus on her and distract her, and the other to carry out the task of washing her.

If bathing is always difficult, you may have to bathe the person less often. Although it's important to keep the person clean, a bath may not be necessary every day. A sponge bath can serve the same purpose as a bath or shower and may be more acceptable to the person, because she can remain partially covered. It's okay to limit bathing to once a week, with sponge baths the other days.

If the person is incontinent, it's especially important to wash the genital area thoroughly, even if it's the only area you clean that day. Always tell the person that you are going to wash their private areas before you do it. Even if only these important parts get washed, the bath is a success.

# When Accidents Happen

Incontinence may begin in Stage 2 or Stage 3 of Alzheimer's disease, depending on the person. There can be medical reasons for incontinence, some of which may be treatable. If the Alzheimer's disease is the only cause of the incontinence, there may still be things you can do to help. At some point, however, you may simply have to accept incontinence as a fact of life with an Alzheimer's patient.

What is most important is your attitude toward the incontinence and the resulting tasks you are faced with in dealing with it. If you are freaked out by having to deal with diapers and accidents, it will upset and agitate the person with AD. If you treat the person as a failure, he or she will feel bad and continue to fail. If you simply accept the problem as part of the disease and treat him or her with respect and sensitivity, both of you are likely to adapt to the incontinence much more easily.

## Why Accidents Happen

There are many possible causes of incontinence in older people besides the brain damage that is a result of Alzheimer's disease. Some of them are …

- Frequent drinking of diuretic-containing fluids, such as coffee, tea, cocoa, beer, or colas.
- Side effects of medications.
- Infections, such as urinary tract infections.
- In men—prostate problems.
- In women—constipation or weak pelvic muscles.
- Anxiety or fear.
- Feeling rushed.

If the person with AD is incontinent and none of these conditions are present, the following AD-related factors could be causing the problem:

- Inability to connect the sensation of needing to go to the bathroom with the process of doing so.

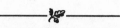

Becoming totally able to handle every aspect of one's personal hygiene takes a newborn baby at least five years. Even then the child may not be allowed to take a bath without supervision. It takes approximately the same amount of time for an adult with Alzheimer's to become totally incontinent. The process begins as the loss of eye-hand coordination causes the person with AD to have trouble managing his or her clothing. It gets worse as the disease causes the loss of the person's rote memory, which is what allows us to carry out activities without consciously thinking through every step. Finally, the disease will severely disrupt the brain's signals to the body and result in the total inability to control the bowel or bladder. Incontinence, therefore, isn't simply about forgetting where the bathroom is—it's a result of progressive brain damage.

---
🍃
---

Most caregivers are initially reluctant to having the person with AD use adult diaper products. Wearing a pad, however, doesn't strip one of one's dignity. People dealing with spinal injuries, Multiple Sclerosis, ALS, cancer, and other illnesses also have to deal with incontinence. Adult diapers are used to keep the affected person clean, to protect clothing and furniture, and to give both the person and the caregiver a reprieve from being near the bathroom at all times.

---

- Inability to express the need to go to the bathroom.
- Inability to find the bathroom, or having too far to go to get there.
- Inability to find the toilet once in the bathroom—it may blend in with white floors and walls.
- Inability to remember what to do once in the bathroom.
- Trouble getting his or her clothes undone.
- Poor lighting in the bathroom or on the way there.
- A bed that is too high or chair that is too soft to get out of quickly.
- Finding the task of going to the bathroom too difficult or requiring too many steps.

## Dealing with Incontinence

Once a person with AD is having more than occasional accidents and you can't find a reason for it other than Alzheimer's disease, you will have to begin to deal with incontinence as a regular part of life. The fear of dealing with incontinence is often far greater than the reality of simply handling it.

Here are some things you can do:

- Learn to recognize the nonverbal cues a person gives about needing to go to the bathroom, and respond to them quickly.
- Schedule frequent visits to the bathroom.
- Recognize that when a person starts to fidget or pick at his or her clothing near the groin, it may signal a need to urinate.
- Look for a pattern of where and when accidents happen.
- Have signs with words and pictures to identify the bathroom.
- Make sure the person's clothes are easy to get on and off.
- Put a commode next to the bed at night.
- Provide adequate lighting to and in the bathroom.
- Decrease the amount of fluids at night to prevent nighttime incontinence.

Many people find it best to deal with incontinence by having the person with AD use adult absorbency pads. If you decide to use them, you can have the affected person wear regular underwear over them, so he or she feels less childlike. Be sure to change incontinence pads often and keep the person's skin clean. Lotions and powders should also be used to protect the skin.

The question for some caregivers is not whether to use adult pads, but how to get the person with Alzheimer's disease to be willing to wear them. The decision to use these products, however, should be your choice, not the affected person's, and the less you make of it, the better. Don't ask for permission to use incontinence pads. Just treat them as simply another part of the dressing routine.

When putting on the pads, it sometimes helps to work from behind the person. Your presence is less obvious that way. Don't say things like: "It's time to change your diaper." Instead, talk about getting freshened-up or changing clothes. You don't have to remind the person of his or her problem. Just be matter-of-fact about the whole thing.

A person with AD who has urinary incontinence may or may not also have bowel incontinence. If the person does have bowel incontinence, make sure it is not due to fecal impaction or drug side effects. Bowel incontinence can sometimes be helped by learning when the person generally has bowel movements and getting him or her to sit on the toilet for a while at that time.

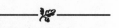

Incontinence isn't necessarily a reason to put the person with AD in a facility. Many caregivers take care of an affected person after he or she becomes incontinent. Your attitude and your willingness to take charge of the situation are important. The first incontinence problems may begin while the person is still able to do many other things. If you see incontinence as simply another symptom of Alzheimer's, you may be able to handle it yourself for quite a while.

# 20

# Time Off: Getting Help for You

❧

What is the most important thing that you can do for yourself if you are the primary caregiver for a person with Alzheimer's disease? The answer—hands down—from those who have been through what you are going through is: "Get time off!" Why is time off so important? After all, if you are the affected person's spouse, you were used to spending most of your time with him or her before the disease. Being a caregiver, however, is a very different role than being a spouse. When you spent time with your spouse before the disease, it was pleasurable and relaxing for you. Now it can often be draining or exhausting.

Time off gives you the chance to nurture yourself with other relationships—your children and friends if you are the affected person's spouse; and your own spouse, significant other, children, and friends if you are the affected person's child. You can't ignore the other people in your life when you are caring for a person with AD. Your role as a caregiver may go on for years. You need your friends and relatives and they need you during this time. Time off also allows you to attend a support group, to take care of business, and to just have some fun—which you deserve to have.

It's critical that you get regular weekly time off to recharge your physical and emotional batteries, and that you take a real break—a vacation—at least once a year. But how do you do it?

Who will watch the person with AD while you are away? In this chapter, you'll learn about some of the options for help that are out there. It's up to you, however, to take advantage of those options.

---

### One Caregiver's Journey

"In my support group, I was surprised that so many of the spouses who were taking care of their partners with Alzheimer's were so reluctant to ask their children for anything. I think they were afraid the children would say no. Before the disease struck, they would ask the children to come and visit them and the children would always say they were too busy. So, when it came time to ask for help, they were afraid they would get the same reaction. They couldn't bear being turned down and disappointed, so they didn't ask. This is too bad because the children might have come through. Especially if the caregiver had just asked the adult child to do something, such as have lunch with him or her."

---

## Help from Family and Friends

The first place that you think of turning for help so you can have time off may be from those closest to you and to the person with AD. Since a child or friend may want to spend time with the affected person anyway, it can be an opportunity for you to get a break. Some relatives and friends, however, may be reluctant to visit the person with AD. They may not understand the disease and feel uncomfortable.

You can help overcome that reluctance by educating them a little about the disease and suggesting specific things they can do with the person with AD. Explain to reluctant relatives or friends what behaviors they can expect and how to react. If the family or friend has a good experience the first time he or she helps, you may be able to count on him or her again.

Some local chapters of the Alzheimer's Association have special sessions to train family members and friends to be visitors. This is great if it's available in your area because it can help your potential helper feel confident and at ease with the person with AD, thus making the visit not only a welcome time off for you, but also a pleasurable experience for the person with AD.

If you have a large extended family, schedule a family meeting from time to time to help other family members understand the situation and to involve them in sharing the caregiving responsibilities. If you tell others that you need time off at least once a week, the group may find a way to help you get it.

It often isn't easy to find the help you need to get time for yourself, but you must keep trying, no matter how difficult it may seem. Reach out beyond your immediate family and try to develop a support system of friends, neighbors, relatives, and professionals who will be resources for you. Make a list of people you know and the support that each one will or might provide in different areas:

- Those who can stay with your loved one for short periods
- Those on whom you can rely for specific tasks and assistance, such as transportation, running an errand, preparing a meal, or shopping
- Those with whom you can share your feelings
- Those with whom you can go out and have a good time
- Those to whom you can go when you need professional help

Make sure you put people on the list in each area who are best suited for giving that specific kind of help. When someone seems willing to provide some regular help in one area, don't take advantage of him or her by asking for other kinds of support. Spread the wealth and you will get more consistent support from others on your list.

Also, don't expect others to ask you if you need help. It is up to you to do the asking. But just in case someone offers, have a list prepared of tasks that need to be done.

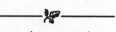

Research on caregiving shows that when a competent caregiver is taking care of an Alzheimer's patient, other family members don't do much to help. Unfortunately, friends don't fill the gaps either. If that is the case in your family, remember that many aspects of care can be performed by someone outside the family—and in some cases, better than what family members would provide. Rather than pressuring a reluctant family member to help take care of the person with AD, ask them to contribute to the cost of professional help.

Paying for outside help to provide you with time off can be expensive. You may be eligible to have a home healthcare aide paid for by Medicare, Medicaid, or some other insurance plan. If not, you may be able to find a volunteer or low-cost organization that can provide help. In Michigan, for example, there is a program called Seniors 4 Seniors that provides such services as cooking, house cleaning, chauffeuring, or companionship for a small fee.

# Help from Outside Providers

At some point, most caregivers do—and should—look for outside help beyond family or friends in order to get time off from care giving. There are a number of community resources available in most areas that you can turn to for help. The first thing you have to do is find out what is available, then decide what you can afford and what will be best for you and the person with AD.

The kinds of help available to you include:

- **Adult Day Care programs.** Programs that provide Alzheimer's patients with the opportunity to interact with others in a supportive environment, usually in a community center or facility. You can generally take the person with AD to an adult day care center for one to five days a week.

- **Companionship services.** Services that provide companions for people in the home. The companion may also offer supervision and personal care.

- **Home health aides.** Professional caregivers who provide personal care to patients at home and assist with light household tasks.

- **Homemaker or housekeeping services.** Services that provide household assistance, including shopping, laundry, cleaning, and meal preparation.

- **Respite care.** Services that provide relief to caregivers by offering short-term, temporary care for patients in the home or in a facility.

- **Skilled nursing care.** Medically oriented care provided by licensed nurses.

# Home Aides—Where to Find Them

If you decide you want to employ someone in your home to help care for the person with AD so you can get some time off, the first decision you must make is whether to hire an agency or directly hire someone yourself.

## Agencies

If you don't have the time, but do have the money, you can hire a case management service for a fee. These are agencies that will provide you with a case manager who will meet with you, assess your needs, and then arrange for the services you need. He or she will find the people you need to work in your home and monitor them to make sure they are fulfilling your needs. The main problem with these services is that they are fairly expensive.

If you decide to forgo the expense of a case manager, you first have to decide what kind of help you need. In the early stages of the disease, simple companionship may be all that is necessary. Later, you may want people to help with personal care. You may also really want someone to help with shopping and preparing food. As the disease progresses, you may need to have medical professionals who know how to take care of a patient confined to the bed.

Second, you have to decide whether to go through an agency or hire the person on your own. A home healthcare agency, a visiting nurse's agency, and a homemaker service are organizations or companies that have lists of people who have been screened by the agency before they are sent out to you. The agency's fee is usually billed by the visit or by the hour.

If you decide to hire someone to work for you through an agency, make sure that it is a licensed and accredited agency. You can check with your local Area Agency on Aging for lists of agencies. If you are eligible for Medicare, you must choose an agency that is certified by Medicare to get reimbursed for services. The same applies to your insurance company or HMO. If they are paying, they usually have lists of approved agencies.

It's also important to find out as much as you can about how the agency screens their staff and what type of training, supervision, and monitoring it provides to its staff.

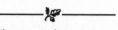

When you do manage to get a break from caregiving, what should you do? You might want to run errands and take care of business matters, but be sure to also plan some fun. See a movie, take a walk in the park, or have lunch with a friend. Although it's not necessarily fun, also use your time off to get a regular checkup from your doctor or dentist. You can't let either your emotional or your physical health deteriorate.

## On Your Own

You will save money by hiring home care aides on your own, but you will have to go through the work of finding applicants and screening them yourself. You will also be the person's employer and will, therefore, be responsible for his or her salary, benefits, firing, and withholding Social Security taxes.

If you decide to hire a person yourself, start the search by talking to family members, doctors, clergy, people in your caregiver support group, and people at senior centers. Also, check with local senior newspapers or magazines and the Area Agency on Aging. If you are looking for a student rather than a professional aide, you could also try the placement offices on college campuses or in nursing and medical schools. If those resources don't provide enough leads, try placing an ad in the local newspaper. You could also post flyers on the bulletin boards at senior centers, hospitals, and colleges.

After posting an ad or getting referrals, first screen your prospective helper on the phone. Ask him or her to tell you about his or her education and previous employment. Explain exactly what you will need—the hours, the days, and the duties. Be sure to ask if the person has had any experience with people with Alzheimer's disease.

If you feel that the person may be right for the position, schedule an interview in your home where you will be able to show him or her around and where he or she will have a chance to meet the person with AD. It might be a good idea to have a friend or family member with you when the applicant comes to your home—it never hurts to have a second opinion. So that it seems formal and professional from the outset, you also might want to buy a standard employment application at your local stationery store for the applicant to fill out.

It's important for you to describe the job in as much detail as possible so that the applicant understands what is expected of him or her. Be specific. Tell him or her the number of hours to be worked, the time to report to work, and the time to leave work. Be sure to mention any unusual information about the person with AD so that the applicant knows exactly what problems to expect.

What are some of the things you should look for in the applicant? You should decide what qualities are most important to you, but as a start, here's a checklist. Does the person ...

- Seem compassionate?
- Communicate effectively?
- Seem gentle and caring?
- Appear cooperative and willing to follow instructions?
- Seem professional and competent?
- Listen well?
- Seem compatible with your loved one?
- Have experience with any special medical or other equipment that he or she may need to use?
- Seem friendly and mature?
- Seem at ease?
- Appear to be in good health and physically able to perform required duties?
- Have a sense of humor?
- Have experience caring for people with Alzheimer's disease?
- Have a valid driver's license if he or she is expected to transport you or your family member?

Make it clear during the interview that you can fire, as well as hire. Make sure the applicant understands what rules and behaviors are unacceptable to you, such as tardiness, not performing job duties, or poor attitude.

Be sure to ask whether or not the applicant feels there are any aspects of the work that he or she isn't capable of or comfortable doing. Provide some examples of difficult behaviors to see how he or she might respond.

Before hiring the applicant, it's absolutely essential that you check all references and previous employment carefully. Also, you might want to check for a criminal record with local law enforcement officials. It's important to make sure the person has not been involved in elder abuse or neglect actions.

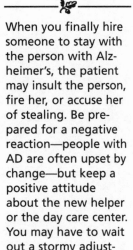

When you finally hire someone to stay with the person with Alzheimer's, the patient may insult the person, fire her, or accuse her of stealing. Be prepared for a negative reaction—people with AD are often upset by change—but keep a positive attitude about the new helper or the day care center. You may have to wait out a stormy adjustment period. Reassure the person that this is a good thing for both of you.

You may or may not want to draw up an agreement or contract with your helper. If you do, it should list the name, address, phone number, social security number, a schedule of days and hours for work, days off, holidays off, services to be performed, and any benefits you agree on. You may need to consult an elder law attorney or your accountant to make sure you withhold the proper taxes and have proper insurance coverage.

## How to Supervise Your Help

Before the new helper is left alone for the first day with the Alzheimer's patient, it might help to provide some orientation for a few days, so the new helper and the person with AD can become acquainted with each other. When you do go out for the first time and each time thereafter, be ready with a written list of instructions so that you can leave the house soon after the helper arrives and won't waste time giving lengthy instructions. If you have a computer, write the instructions on it so you can change them as new behaviors and information arise.

In addition to providing basic information about the person's schedule and where things are, also give the aide some tips that will help him or her take care of the person with AD. For example, if the affected person has a favorite towel for bath time or likes to sit in a particular spot while eating lunch, write these extra tips in your instructions.

Be sure to give your helper emergency numbers—for the doctor, neighbors, other family members, the local pharmacist, and, of course, your cell phone or pager number. If the person is a home healthcare aide who will also be providing housekeeping services, be sure to include a detailed list of tasks you want him or her to perform and where the necessary supplies are located. If the same aide comes each week, make sure you keep supplies in the same place and that there is an adequate supply.

Remember, it's your responsibility to oversee and supervise the people you hire. It's up to you to direct them and to give them feedback when things aren't what you want. It's also important to praise their work from time to time.

## Adult Day Care

Instead of, or in addition to, hiring helpers in your home, most communities have Adult Day Care centers where you can take the person with Alzheimer's. These centers provide an opportunity for him or her to socialize with others and engage in various recreational and support activities in a supervised group setting. Many people with AD enjoy these programs immensely—they give him or her a break from staying home all the time and a chance to interact with other people besides you. And, of course, you get the whole day off.

Adult Day Care centers are offered by hospitals, senior community centers, and private organizations. The services are generally for frail, mentally and otherwise impaired adults. In the best of these centers, the goal is not just to be a place where the affected individual can be left for the day, but to help to maintain or even improve the level of functioning as long as possible and delay further deterioration.

Although it varies among different centers, some of the activities and services that Adult Day Care centers offer include …

- General care and supervision.
- Meals and snacks, including special diets.
- Exercise.
- Assistance with activities of daily living and personal care, including eating, walking, toileting, bathing, shampooing, and shaving.
- Group social activities, such as games, arts and crafts, music, singing, and dancing.
- Recreational outings.
- Reminiscence and intergenerational experiences.
- Special activities, such as gardening and playing with pets.
- Health monitoring, including blood pressure, food or liquid intake, weight, podiatrist visits, and assistance with medication.

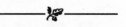

Once you have someone taking care of the person with AD, you need to be sure that you use your time off efficiently. To do that, plan in advance by making a list of the tasks that you need to do outside the house. Then, plan your errands according to where the shops are or how important the errand is so you can get everything you need to do accomplished.

- Transportation—some centers will pick up and drop off the person with AD.
- Counseling and physical, occupational, and speech therapy.

Don't be discouraged by your first visit to an Adult Day Care center. You may be upset at seeing other people with AD or frail elderly people, and feel that they are more impaired than your loved one. The other people may be interesting to the person with AD, however. He or she may enjoy helping others who are more impaired.

If an Adult Day Care center sounds good to you, how do you choose the right center? First, get a list of centers from the local Alzheimer's Association or by calling the National Respite Locator Service at 1-800-773-5433. Call each center that seems convenient to you and have them send you information.

The information should include the center's eligibility criteria and conditions accepted; staff credentials; number of staff per participant; a list of the daily and monthly activities for patients; information about the meals they provide, including sample menus; information about the sponsoring agency or owner of the center, including whether it is for-profit or not-for-profit; the hours of operation and days open; whether or not transportation is offered; the application procedures and the cost; and whether or not there is the possibility of financial assistance.

After you've narrowed down the choices based on the information you received, make an appointment to visit the centers that seem like they might work for you. How does the place look to you? Is it clean and free of unpleasant odors? Do the participants seem as though they are enjoying themselves? Is the staff friendly and competent? Is the facility comfortable, and does it include a place for patients to lie down when tired?

When you've chosen the best center, try it out for a few days. It may take several visits for your loved one to feel comfortable in a new setting and with a new routine. Remember also that the person with AD may not be able to recall all the activities he or she enjoyed during the day, so ask the staff how he or she did.

Once the routine is established, you can relax and take care of yourself, knowing that your loved one is having a good time and being well-cared-for.

## Vacations: Short-Term Respite Care

We all need regular vacations from our work and our daily lives. As a caregiver, that is especially the case. Don't let a year go by without taking a vacation from caregiving. But how do you manage to take a vacation? Short-term respite care or short-stay residential care is available in your community for just that purpose. Hospitals, nursing homes, and, particularly, residential care homes offer families the opportunity to place older relatives in their facilities for short stays—a weekend, a week, or a few weeks. The National Respite Locator Service, your doctor, or the Area Agency on Aging can assist with referrals and arrangements.

It's important for you to take a vacation before your stress level gets too high. Are you hesitant to use short-term care to take a vacation out of fear that once you stop caregiving, even for a short period, you won't be able to do it again? Relax; you will be able to return to the work of caregiving—refreshed and relaxed—just as you always returned to a job after a vacation or to school after summer vacation.

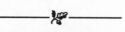

Many Adult Day Care centers also offer services for you, the caregiver. Some of the common services offered include caregiver support groups, care or case management services, information and referrals, literature on Alzheimer's disease, other medical information, seminars on a variety of care issues, medical equipment, clothing catalogues, newsletters, and brochures with tips on managing difficult behaviors. You may have found the place for one-stop shopping for all of your caregiving needs.

# 21

# Moving the Patient in Advance of a Crisis

Approximately one third of Alzheimer's patients are taken care of in a facility outside the home and—because so many people in this country have Alzheimer's disease—about 60 percent of all nursing home patients are people with AD. There are a number of reasons that Alzheimer's patients live in nursing homes or other facilities. Sometimes the AD patient has no family member able to care for him or her. The affected person may have no living spouse, and his or her children may not live in the same city or may have too many responsibilities to take on the task of full-time caregiving. Sometimes the family member who has been caring for the person with AD is no longer able to handle the task. Sometimes, the family has simply decided that institutional care is better than the care family members could provide.

Whatever the reason for the decision to move an AD patient to a facility, it is often a painful one for the caregiver and the family. Rather than seeing the move to an institution as simply the next phase of care for the person with AD, caregivers and family often feel guilty and defeated by the decision. Putting someone in an institution—even someone who can no longer care for himself—breaks the unspoken promises that family members have made to one another. It makes us feel as though we are disloyal or ungrateful to those who have loved and supported us.

Because the decision to put a person with AD into a facility is so fraught with negative feelings, it's important to make the decision carefully and in advance of a crisis. In this chapter, we'll explore how to go about making the decision, so that you can be sure you are doing what is best for you and for the person with AD.

*One Caregiver's Journey*

"When I led Alzheimer's support groups, I used to take my groups to visit nursing homes. The people in my groups were usually afraid of them. The idea of placement was very scary. There were a couple of good places I knew about and wanted to show to the caregivers. I wanted them to know that if things got so bad that they couldn't take it, there were places that were nice, where they could feel comfortable placing their loved one with AD. Even if you never end up placing the person in a nursing home, if you at least know that you have an option, it can be a relief."

## When Is the Right Time?

When it comes to putting someone you love into an institution, you may feel like there is never a right time. There is, however, a wrong time. The wrong time is in the middle of a crisis or an emergency, when you have not had the time to plan for the move or when you are too upset to make the best decisions. If you have been taking care of the person with AD—whether in your home or with a hired caretaker in an assisted-living situation—you have invested a great deal of yourself in providing care. When you can no longer provide the best care, you will want to feel that the place you put the person is the best possible choice. To be assured of that, you need to investigate possible facilities in advance of a crisis.

What kind of crisis might occur? The person with AD might be admitted to a hospital for some urgent reason—a broken hip, pneumonia, a stroke, or any number of reasons. You might feel, or the doctor might tell you, that you won't be able to care for the person at home any longer and a nursing home is the best place for him or her. Then, in a panic, you must find a suitable home. You will have to choose a place that has a bed immediately available, and you won't have time to think about what you want or need from the nursing home setting. You certainly won't have much time to get your feelings sorted out.

Instead of waiting for an emergency or crisis to force you to place the person in a facility, at the first moment you realize that some sort of placement may be necessary or best for the person with AD in the future, begin to think about the issue and begin planning for the move.

If you take time to select a home that you can afford and that is best for the person with AD, then, when the time comes to move him or her, you will be ready. Once you have prepared for it, the move will be smoother—whether it is from your home or from the hospital.

## The Right Time for You

One of the main things to consider when thinking about the time to move a person with AD to a facility is your own physical, emotional, and spiritual health. How much care is too much for you? You may burn yourself out from the stresses of taking care of the person with AD. You may become physically sick or emotionally overwrought. Read Chapter 25, "The Present: Caring for Yourself Through It All," to help evaluate whether or not you are showing signs of caregiver stress. If you are, either seriously start taking better care of yourself or begin accepting that you are going to have to put the person in a facility—or both.

For some of us, it is the emotional burden of watching the progression of the disease that is too much. When the person no longer recognizes you, it may be too hard for you to continue to care for him or her day after day and night after night. You may be so emotionally upset by the disease and by your overwhelming responsibilities that you snap at the person with AD or burst into tears frequently.

For others, including many of those who are older, the physical stamina required to help the person dress, bathe, and

Placing a person in a nursing home is difficult. An unplanned placement makes it harder for you to achieve the confidence and trust in the new facility that will make the change easier emotionally. You need to know that the home can provide the kind of care you want for the person and that it will allow you to retain the kind of caregiving role you want with the person. To be assured of both, plan the move in advance.

Caregivers should know that there are a number of legal duties or liabilities that come with the job of caregiving. In most states, caregivers are bound by elder abuse laws not to abuse the elderly person (physically, mentally, or monetarily), and to report any incidents of abuse or suspected abuse. Caregivers must also provide a clean and safe environment, nutritious meals, and clean bedding and clothes. Those who are in charge of the elderly person's finances must use that money properly, purchasing necessary services for the benefit of the person to whom care is given. Failure to provide care, failure to get care, and failure to purchase care are all forms of abuse or neglect.

move around—while also doing all the household chores—may simply be too much. Even with hired household or medical help, the demands may be so great that you go to bed utterly exhausted every night and never wake up rested enough.

For still others, it is the spiritual angst you feel. You may not feel that your life is worth living. You feel tied to the home with a person who no longer either recognizes you or seems to love you. There is nothing in your life that gives you any pleasure or any hope. You are no longer the life-loving optimistic person you once were. A smile rarely crosses your face.

If you see yourself as physically, emotionally, or spiritually unhealthy, be willing to consider that continuing the role of primary caregiver may not be for you.

Caregiving is a serious responsibility, and many people who feel they can handle it ultimately realize that they can't. To protect older people from abuse at the hands of caregivers, many states have passed elder abuse laws. Even a well-meaning caregiver can become so stressed that he or she yells at the AD patient or withholds affection. You must accept the physical, psychological, and legal duties to provide the necessary care. If you are reaching a point where you are no longer able to provide the proper care physically or emotionally, it's time to consider placement of the patient in a facility.

The job of a full-time caregiver is much too strenuous and stressful for most people to endure forever. You need to be honest with yourself and admit when you have reached your limit. Admit to yourself: "I am not able to do this anymore." If you feel relief at saying those words, stop, research alternatives, get help from others, and know that you are doing the right thing.

## The Right Time for the Alzheimer's Patient

The truth is that many Alzheimer's patients do better in a structured environment with trained professionals than they do in their own homes. For one thing, the environment often offers more opportunity for stimulation than at home. The affected person can share meals and planned activities with other patients instead of sitting at home watching television while you are busy with household duties.

In other cases, the patient simply may not have someone who can afford the time to be a primary caregiver. Perhaps he or she is at home with a full-time home healthcare provider. Is that really better than being in an environment with other patients with whom he or she can socialize?

In other instances, the patient may be almost bedridden. Even though you have taken care of the affected person through the other phases of the disease, this final stage may be much more challenging. You have to learn how to prevent pressure sores. You have to feed the person so he or she doesn't choke. Medical professionals who have been trained to deal with these issues may provide better care for the person with AD than you can.

## Involve Others in the Decision

The decisions of whether to place your loved one in a facility, and when and where to place him, are too important to make on your own. It's essential that you consult with your doctor, with everyone in the family, and even with the person with AD, depending on his or her ability to understand the discussion.

### Medical Professionals

Your doctor should be consulted if you are thinking about placing the person with AD in a facility. The doctor knows the person with AD and knows his or her level of functioning and thus may be able to make a referral to the type of facility that offers the best level of care. (See the following sections for the different levels of care that facilities offer.) Even more important than the doctor's referral is the fact that he or she may be able to reassure you that you are making the right decision or help the family come to a decision if there are those who are ambivalent about or opposed to moving the person with AD to a home.

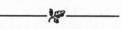

You may feel that you should care for your loved one at home no matter what the cost. The cost, however, is not yours alone. Your other relationships suffer when you are overburdened. And the Alzheimer's patient also pays a price—she loses the opportunity for social contact. She may never understand that and may never agree with your decision. Nevertheless, you still must be the one to make the decision based on what is best for both of you.

If your doctor has not been that involved with the person with AD, or is not that familiar with AD care, you might instead seek the help of other medical professionals, such as social workers, counselors, or nurses. Many hospitals have social workers on staff who can help you think about this issue. If you call the local Alzheimer's Association, they may be able to refer you to professionals who can help you make this decision.

## Family Members

Everyone in the family should be involved in the decision to place the person with Alzheimer's disease in a facility, even if the caregiving has been left to only one member of the family. If every family member is initially consulted and has a chance to offer his or her input, the ultimate placement is likely to go more smoothly. If a family member has not been consulted, he or she may be upset and there can be tension in the family, which no one needs—particularly with all the stress of taking care of the person with AD.

Sometimes, a family member who hasn't been taking care of the person with AD will be supportive of the move to a facility because it will ease his or her guilt at not being there on a day-to-day basis. Other times, a family member who hasn't been very involved will oppose the placement. Even though it may irritate you, take the time to try to educate the person about the disease and explain the stresses of caregiving. If you are patient, he or she will probably come around to your point of view.

### One Caregiver's Journey

"My brother was not close to my mother. He had a terrible argument with her before she was diagnosed with Alzheimer's over something she said to his daughter. So, he was totally delighted that I was taking care of her. I used to call him if I had to make an important decision, such as when I decided it was time to place her in a facility. I didn't want all of the responsibility. He always went along with me, but it was good to have someone with whom I could talk things over."

## Involve the Person with Alzheimer's

Even under the best of circumstances, it's not an easy decision to place your loved one with AD in a home; but the decision is even harder when he or she has made you promise never to put him or her in a facility, and remains opposed to the placement.

There are many reasons why someone with AD—or anyone—would never want to be in a nursing home or other facility. The affected person may feel afraid of being abandoned by you or afraid of being mistreated or abused in the home. He or she may know of someone else who was mistreated in a home.

What should you do if you have made a promise not to put the person in a home, but now you feel that circumstances make it unavoidable? Of course, it's best not to make that promise in the first place—and chances are that now the person with AD won't remember the promise anyway. If the person with AD does remember your promise and is upset about the idea of moving to a home, try to reassure him that you will never abandon him and will always protect him. Promise that you will always provide him with the best care you can afford and that you are only doing what you feel is best for him and for the rest of the family. And promise that you will always see that he is treated with respect and dignity.

If you take time to patiently talk about the issue with the person with AD, he may eventually understand that you are doing what you must and that you are not abandoning him.

## Allow Time to Find the Right Place

Finding the right facility can be a difficult process. There are so many things to take into consideration—the right location, an affordable price, and, of course, most importantly, the facility that will provide the best care. (See Chapter 22, "How to Choose the Right Nursing Home.") Also, most decent facilities that offer long-term care to Alzheimer's and other patients have waiting lists. In some cases, the waiting list may be as long as a year or two. Therefore, it's very important to start early in your search for a facility for the person with AD.

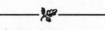

In determining whether it's the right time to place the person with AD in a facility, you might ask yourself several key questions. The first is whether or not the patient would benefit from the social activities provided by the placement. The second is whether or not he or she would even be likely to recognize a change in the environment. And finally, of course, is whether or not care is needed beyond your capacity.

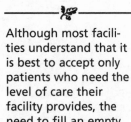

Although most facilities understand that it is best to accept only patients who need the level of care their facility provides, the need to fill an empty apartment or bed might induce them to accept people who are not right for them. Therefore, it's a good idea to call a reputable, state-licensed referral agency to help you find the proper facility. See Appendix C for listings of referral agencies or call your local Alzheimer's Association.

The first decision you have to make is what level and type of facility is best for the person with AD. Often, families will place an Alzheimer's patient at the wrong level, either in a facility that is designed to care for people who require more serious medical care than the person with AD needs, or in a facility that doesn't have the necessary medical and support services required to meet his or her needs.

Your doctor can be your best ally in finding a facility that is right for your loved one. He or she can help you assess the level of care the person with AD needs and will be able to give the affected person a complete physical exam, which most facilities require.

Although the names vary from state to state, generally speaking, there are four types of care facilities that can provide the type of care an Alzheimer's patient requires:

- Retirement residences with assisted-living programs
- Small, licensed residential care homes
- Dedicated Alzheimer's care facilities
- Nursing homes

## Retirement Residence with Assisted-Living Program

Most retirement homes have licensed personal care programs that are appropriate for those in the early stages of Alzheimer's disease when the most common problem is short-term memory loss and intermittent confusion. Some of these facilities have special programs for people with dementia or AD that emphasize a more social approach to care. As the disease progresses and care needs increase or behavior becomes extreme, patients are generally moved from these types of facilities to one dedicated to working with dementia patients, or to a nursing home.

## Licensed Residential Care Home

These facilities are also called "homes for the aged" or "personal care homes" in some states. They are mostly small, licensed group homes that provide a room, meals, supervision, and some other assistance. They typically have six or fewer residents. Their fees vary widely and, when they cater to AD patients, they are appropriate for people in the middle or advanced stages of the disease. There are no federal standards for these facilities, and state regulations vary immensely. If you use such a program, you need to get a good recommendation from a reliable source and then monitor it carefully to make sure the quality of care is good.

### One Caregiver's Journey

"When I placed my mother in the small, six-bed facility, I asked the owner how he got people with Alzheimer's to do things like go to the bathroom. I couldn't get my mother to use the toilet or to even change her underwear, and neither could the aide I hired to take care of her. He said, 'Well, we have our ways. We learn how to do it with each person.' He would do things like distract her and use humor. He was very understanding. I was very impressed with the care. And, of course, they never hurt anyone. I would drop in at various times and she never had any bruises."

## Alzheimer's Dedicated Care Facility

These facilities may be harder to find and can be quite costly. They are appropriate for people in the advanced stages of the disease or those whose behavior is quite unpredictable. They are usually not nursing homes, but are licensed as residential care facilities. The accommodations tend to be more institution-like than the homes for the aged or residential care homes, and usually residents are housed two to a room. What differentiates this type of facility from simply a residential care home or nursing home is that only dementia patients are accepted into the facility. Also, the care is specifically designed to make residents feel comfortable and secure. The staff in these facilities is often better trained than those in the average nursing or residential home, and has more experience in working with Alzheimer's patients.

Most families only choose a nursing home as a last resort, because nursing homes are essentially medical institutions. They look like institutions, and patients are treated as patients, not residents. There is little or no privacy; each patient must share a tiny room with only a drawn curtain to divide his or her space from the other patients in the room. Very sick and bedridden patients are housed with those who are still mobile.

## Nursing Home with a Dedicated Alzheimer's Care Program

A nursing home is appropriate for those in the advanced and terminal stages of Alzheimer's disease in which severe physical and mental deterioration has taken place. Many nursing homes have a special wing of their facilities dedicated to Alzheimer's care.

In most states, nursing homes are considered healthcare facilities and, as such, are licensed and scrutinized by the state health department. As medical facilities, they are allowed to provide services that cannot be dispensed in assisted-living or residential care homes. Typically, these services involve managing potentially serious medical problems, such as infections, wound care, IV therapy, and care for those who are bedridden and are unable to do anything on their own.

Since the advent of HMOs and managed care, hospitals have been discharging patients who are sick to nursing homes much earlier than they have in the past. These patients may need highly skilled care similar to what hospital patients receive. AD patients, however, have different needs—they need a nice environment and increasing amounts of personal care. They may make heavy demands on the nursing-aide staff because of their unpredictable behavior. That is why, if possible, other types of facilities are generally better for AD patients unless the person is in the terminal stage of the disease.

As you can see, just deciding which level of care and which type of facility you feel is best for the person with AD will take some time. After you have narrowed it down, there are still numerous other decisions you must make (which the next chapter covers). This is why you must start planning early and allow yourself adequate time to find the right place for your loved one with AD.

# 22

# How to Choose the Right Nursing Home

In the United States there are over 17,000 nursing homes with more than 1.5 million residents. In the next few decades, three out of five people over the age of 65 will need some type of long-term care, and the number of people living in nursing homes is expected to reach five million.

With a growing number of choices and increasing competition for the best homes, how do you find the right facility for your loved one with Alzheimer's? Choosing a good facility involves doing some research to make an informed decision. As many as one out of four nursing homes each year are cited for causing serious injury or death to a resident, so finding a good facility is essential. To do so, you must carefully evaluate the possible facilities. The guidelines in this chapter will help you find and choose a facility that offers the safest and best environment for your loved one with Alzheimer's.

———— 🦋 ————

The best place to find information on long-term-care facilities is through referrals or recommendations from doctors, home care professionals, geriatric care managers, social workers, friends, and clergy. You can also check through the Eldercare Locator, your state or local health department, the department of aging, and your local Alzheimer's Association. For additional help, you can seek out the ombudsperson service in your state—a free service that helps families find the right facility to suit their individual needs.

# The Level of Care Needed

The first decision you must make is the level of care that is right for the person with AD. You may want your loved one to live in a retirement residence with an assisted-living program, a small licensed residential care home, a dedicated Alzheimer care facility or a nursing home, depending on the stage of the disease and the level of care needed.

If you are considering a nursing home, you must decide whether or not the person with AD requires skilled care or custodial care. Skilled care is necessary only if the Alzheimer's patient has a disease or injury that needs ongoing treatment. Patients in the final stage of Alzheimer's often need skilled care. Most patients in the earlier stages of Alzheimer's disease require custodial care. This type of care usually includes assistance with most activities of daily living, such as eating, dressing, bathing, medication management, and walking.

Some nursing homes have designated Alzheimer's or dementia units, but the kind of care included in such units may vary a great deal. Some units may have precautions for those who wander, special training for staff in dealing with difficult behaviors, activities geared for those with memory loss, and additional special features. Other facilities may simply house the AD patients together. If you are thinking of placing your loved one in a special unit, ask what makes it special.

# Geographical Area

After you have narrowed down your choices by the kind of facility and the level of care, location becomes the next important factor. You will probably want a facility that is reasonably close to your home to make visiting easier. Your loved one may live in a nursing home for several years and, if it's too far away, it may be difficult for you to visit as often as you would like to. A good facility a few miles away might be better in the long run than a great facility that requires a drive of an hour or two.

Don't minimize the importance of a convenient location. Frequent visits may not only be a comfort to you and other members of the family, it will also give you more opportunities to monitor the care that is being provided. You will be able to form relationships with the staff that will ultimately benefit your loved one. Sometimes, because of long waiting lists or high costs, you may have difficulty finding a facility that is close to you, but don't give up. You might consider temporarily moving your loved one to a facility that is farther away while you wait for a bed at a closer facility.

## Licensing or Certification

Nearly all nursing homes and other care facilities have some form of certification from your state, usually so they can receive Medicaid and Medicare funds. Close to three quarters of all nursing homes are certified by both Medicare and Medicaid. Find out if the facility you are considering is licensed and accredited.

It's best to seek a licensed facility to help protect against abuse or exploitation. Be sure to ask to see a copy of the license. Also, get a copy of the last inspection report for the facility. Check the facility's record with local and state regulatory agencies. A stellar record is great, of course, but a facility that has had a few black marks may still be good. If there were problems in the past, ask if the administration has changed since they were discovered or how the problems were dealt with.

## Financial Considerations

Before you start inspecting facilities, you might also want to narrow down your list by cost. The cost of nursing homes and other long-term care facilities varies, depending on the facility, the part of the country, and the type of care being provided. The average cost nationally is $42,000 per year. This cost will have to be paid by you, by the estate of the person with Alzheimer's disease, by state Medicaid programs, and, to a much smaller extent, by Medicare and other insurance plans. Chapter 6, "Plans for the Future," discusses the important issue of planning ahead for the cost of caring for the person with AD. By now, you probably know whether or not you are eligible for any government program or insurance to pay for the cost of care and, if not, have budgeted the potential cost.

It's a good idea to do a complete background check on the facility, including the owner-ship, management, financial stability, and staff qualifications. You can check with the Chamber of Commerce, the Better Business Bureau, and your state department of health, or use the services of an ombuds-person. As an advocate for residents, an om-budsperson can help you find out about past complaints and lawsuits against the nursing home.

—————— ❧ ——————

The cost of long-term care can be a deceptive issue. As the price gets higher, the amenities of the facility may get better, but the care may not necessarily be any better. A nice lobby with decent art on the walls and plush carpeting doesn't guarantee quality care. In fact, as regulatory agencies will tell you, some of the worst care can be found in some of the very expensive, well-maintained facilities.

To find out the financial costs involved in the facilities you are considering, ask a lot of questions on the phone prior to a visit. Here are a few suggested questions:

- Is the fee daily or monthly, and how much is it?
- What is included and what is not included in the base fee?
- What services are available for extra charges?
- Are fee increases possible?
- What is the policy regarding daily or monthly rate increases?
- When was the last increase?
- How much notice is given before an increase?
- Under what conditions are refunds available to the resident? How much notice is needed?
- Does the facility work with Medicare? Medicaid? Long-term-care insurers? The Veterans Administration?
- How are extra needs met?
- What payment options are available?
- What types of financial arrangements do they accept?
- How long does the facility hold a room if a resident needs hospitalization?

Unfortunately, the choice of which facility to place your loved one with Alzheimer's in is often dictated by economics. If you're on a limited budget and cannot afford $3,000 to $5,000 a month for 24-hour care or $1,500 to $3,000 for residential care, you may have to place the person with AD in a nursing home that accepts your state's Medicaid program.

If the person with AD is initially placed in a facility because of injury or an illness, Medicare will only pay for the room while the person is receiving actual medical services for up to 100 days. Also, no matter what the person's needs, Medicare will only pay for the first 20 days of skilled care.

Although long-term-care insurance and a few health insurance policies will pay for nursing home care, the cost is usually paid by the family until their resources are exhausted and they are eligible for Medicaid. Over 50 percent of the patients in nursing homes are receiving aid from state Medicaid programs. The patient must meet income and resource requirements, although for couples there are provisions under the law to provide some protection for the spouse of the patient. Often, patients will enter care facilities as private-pay patients, but when their resources are "spent down" they apply for Medicaid. Facilities often ask detailed financial questions on the admissions application to ascertain how long the patient can pay privately before needing to apply for Medicaid.

## Inspect the Facility

Once you have made a list of the facilities you are considering, it's important to visit all of them in order to make an informed choice. You may want to visit your top choices more than once, at different times, to observe the routine of the home and really get a sense of the place. Visit all facilities unannounced and try to do so outside of normal visiting hours.

Since you have many things to do during your visit, it will be more productive if you write down the questions you want to ask and carry your checklist with you during the visit. Don't be afraid to take notes while looking around and talking to people.

In general, your visit should include ...

- Looking closely at the building and grounds.
- Talking to some residents.
- Talking to the facility administrator who is in charge of daily operations.
- Talking to other staff members.
- Obtaining a copy of the Admission Agreement.
- Obtaining a copy of the Resident's Bill of Rights. Under Federal law, all nursing homes must have a written description of the rights of the residents, and it must be made available to the resident or family member who requests it.
- Looking for any bruises on the faces, arms, or legs of residents.

Make sure you get all the information about fees in writing. And before you sign any contract, make sure you go over it with an attorney. Even the most wonderful facility administrator is an advocate for the nursing home. You need an advocate for you and your loved one. Also, don't be afraid to keep asking questions. Even after your loved one has moved in, continue to raise any issues that come up.

—————— ❧ ——————

Use your nose when you inspect a facility. Are there odors in the hallways and communal areas? Or is a high level of hygiene maintained throughout the facility? Also, check out a facility like you would any new home. Have needed repairs been made to walls, handrails, flooring, toilets, sinks, showers, electrical outlets, lights, boilers, air-conditioning, special beds, and other equipment? If there are many broken items, it's a good indication that the facility is not run well.

——————————————

- Observing how residents are dressed.
- Observing how residents are occupied—are they wandering aimlessly in the halls or left sitting all alone?
- Observing whether or not calls for assistance are promptly answered both during the day and at night.

During your inspection, look at the quality and condition of the furnishings, and notice whether personal possessions have been brought from home. To get an idea of the physical, emotional, and mental status of the residents, talk to them and their visitors to see if they're satisfied with the conditions.

## Physical Layout

Be sure to focus on the physical layout of the facility. Is it attractive? Is it well-organized? Is it designed for the privacy needs of the patient? Are there safe areas and gardens outside for walking and sitting? What are the dining rooms and community areas like?

Are all entrances, exits, rooms, hallways, and elevators wheelchair and walker accessible? Are exits well-marked? Are the floors slippery? Are floors, sidewalks, and ramps smooth to prevent tripping and falling?

People with Alzheimer's disease also often become confused and agitated in long corridors with dozens of identical-looking doors. Are there individualized doors with distinctive colors and personal touches?

## Residents' Rooms

The look and feel of the residents' rooms is very important in deciding upon a facility. How are they furnished? Are they warm and comforting? To what extent can personal items and furnishings be brought in to create a familiar and comfortable room? Is there a locked space for the Alzheimer's patient's personal belongings? Since people with AD will often walk into other people's rooms and take things out of closets and drawers, how is the theft of personal possessions handled?

Does each room have an emergency system to call for help? If patients share rooms with other residents, how are problems handled? Are heating and air-conditioning systems adequate and working properly? Does the resident have individual control of the heating and cooling systems in his room? How are the resident's personal laundry needs handled? How frequent are linens changed?

## Bathrooms

Does each room have its own bathroom? Does the bathroom have the proper handrails, grab bars, emergency pull-cords, and accessories your loved one will need? How accessible are the bathrooms outside the patient's room? In the later stages of the disease, a private bathroom may not be necessary because the staff must take the AD patient to the bathroom.

In facilities where many residents are likely to be incontinent, bathroom odors are almost inevitable—but they should not be overpowering. How does the staff deal with incontinence? Catheters should be a last resort. Only very few people should have catheter bags attached to their beds or wheelchairs.

## The Staff

Ask if the staff is trained to deal with people who have Alzheimer's. Talk with some of the nurses and ask how they would deal with the types of problems your loved one has. If it is not a facility devoted exclusively to Alzheimer's disease, find out what percent of residents have Alzheimer's. You will definitely want a facility where the staff has experience in dealing with the disease.

Notice the resident-to-staff ratio. The lower the ratio, the better the care in most cases, but the number of staff is also not the only consideration. Is the staff sitting at the nurse's station or are they involved with the residents? Pay attention to how the staff, including the nurse's aides, interact with the residents, particularly with other Alzheimer's patients.

Talk with staff members about the person with AD. An administrator, nurse, or nurse's aide who inquires about your loved one's likes and dislikes, abilities, and problems will probably provide better, more individualized care than a staff member who only talks about policies and procedures.

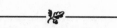

Make sure that the person with AD has the same kind of comforts he or she had at home. For example, if he enjoys watching TV or listening to the radio in the comfort of his room—or is bedridden—are there a television and radio in the room, or can you bring some in? In the later stages of the disease, these types of amenities may not be necessary for your loved one with AD, although they may enable family members to feel better about the placement.

---

**❧**

Find out what kind of nursing staff works at the facility. Nurses' aides generally help residents with daily living activities, such as bathing and dressing. They make beds, serve meals, and provide general patient comforts. Licensed Professional Nurses (LPNs) provide routine medications and any necessary medical treatments ordered by the patient's doctor. In large facilities, nursing services are usually supervised by Registered Nurses (RNs). Find out if an RN or LPN is on each shift.

---

Is the staff welcoming and responsive? How do staff interact with one another? Try to determine the rate of turnover of staff at the facility. A low turnover and happy, satisfied staff members are a good indication of a well-run facility.

## One Caregiver's Journey

"I ended up putting my mother in a six-bed board and care facility rather than a large nursing home. I had heard about this facility from two people in my support group who had their husbands in this small facility. They were absolutely in love with the owner of the place. He was warm and wonderful and was on the premises all the time. It was very well-managed. So, I decided to put my mother in there also. When he sold the place, however, it went downhill. So, I moved her and, at the end, she was at a different place. If you put someone in one of these small facilities, it must be a place where the owner is on the premises all the time. If the owner isn't around, it will be terrible."

## Medical Policies

You will need to find out how routine medical and dental care are handled at the facilities you are considering. Do physicians visit the facility regularly? Does your doctor work with this facility? If not, how experienced are the staff physicians in the care of Alzheimer's patients? If your doctor doesn't practice in the facility you are considering, ask him or her for feedback on the physicians who do practice there.

In some facilities, residents are taken to physicians and dentists. Can they be taken to their own providers? What happens if there is a medical emergency? Is there a physician on call at all times? Which hospital does the facility use? Will the home take the patient to the hospital from the facility if needed? Will the hospital be able to provide the care that your loved one might need? Don't forget to frankly discuss end-of-life decisions. If your loved one has a living will and does not wish to be kept alive with heroic, technological measures, will those wishes be respected? What documents are required?

In many larger facilities, health professionals provide special medical and rehabilitative services for those who need them. Some of the services may or may not be helpful to the AD patient, depending on the stage of the disease. The types of services include physical therapy; occupational therapy, which helps people relearn ways to accomplish daily living tasks, such as bathing, dressing, and eating; speech therapy, which helps the patient to communicate, troubleshoots and treats swallowing disorders, and helps to increase the ability to take in nourishment; respiratory therapy, which helps to treat breathing disorders so that residents are more comfortable and can be more productive in their daily routines; and counseling services, to provide psychological support to residents. Other health professionals who may frequent the nursing home include social workers, podiatrists, eye doctors, dentists, and x-ray technicians.

## General Policies and Considerations

After you have inspected the facility carefully, meet with the administrator to go over questions you may have and find out about general policies. No question is too small or unimportant. You will be paying a lot of money to the place you choose, so you deserve to have all of your concerns answered. Some questions include …

- Are personal services available, such as hair cutting, washing, and tailoring?
- Are pets allowed, and how is it handled if they are?
- Is smoking allowed and, if so, how is it regulated?
- Is someone responsible for shopping for the personal needs of the resident—or is the family responsible for such tasks?
- How is cash handled for the resident's incidental needs?
- Is there a family council that meets to handle complaints?
- How often are families informed of the status of the residents?

———————❦———————

Despite what some facility administrators may claim, it's possible to have a restraint-free environment without an increase in injuries. Also, research confirms that nonrestrained residents require fewer minutes of direct nursing care than similar residents who are restrained. In order to be effective, however, restraint reduction activities need the cooperation of all of the staff of the facility, from the administrators to the nursing assistants and housekeeping personnel.

- Are there periodic meetings scheduled between the staff and each of the families?
- What grounds are cause for the contract to be canceled?

Federal law requires that nursing homes have individual care plans worked out for each resident. Ask the administrator to tell you who develops the plan. Can you participate? As your loved one's Alzheimer's disease progresses, how will the care plan change?

## Safety and Emergency Policies

Of the 1.5 million nursing home residents nationwide, about 50 percent fall at least once each year. Ten to twenty percent of nursing home falls result in serious injuries. Among people 85 years and older, 20 percent of fall-related deaths occur in nursing homes. Find out what safety precautions are in place, particularly for AD patients who might wander and subsequently fall.

Ask about smoke detectors, fire alarms, fire extinguishers, and the evacuation plan. Facilities should have all precautions in working order, along with periodic fire drills. In areas where tornadoes, hurricanes, flooding, or earthquakes might strike, facilities should have a disaster plan. If there have been natural disasters recently, investigate how the facility and its residents fared.

## Visiting Policies

Be sure to check the visiting hours and policies. When can you visit your loved one? How do the visiting hours fit into your schedule? Can you have any privacy with the resident? Can you take the resident off the grounds? The more open and relaxed the facility is about visitors, the better. Facilities that severely restrict visitation might be perfectly fine, but then again, they might have something they wish to hide from visitors.

## Use of Physical and Chemical Restraints

The Nursing Home Reform Act of 1987 states that residents have the right to be free from physical or chemical restraints imposed for purposes of discipline or convenience and not required to treat the resident's medical symptoms. You should find out the facility's policy on the use of restraints—both physical restraints and medications used in behavioral management. Look around and see how many residents are restrained. Be wary of any home in which more than a few residents are restrained or seem overmedicated.

To discover how often restraints are used in a facility, ask how certain behavior problems are generally handled. Has the administration developed written guidelines for handling behavior problems? Under what circumstances are residents medicated?

Though restraints are supposed to help prevent accidents, the use of them may, in fact, cause serious injury. Physical restraints may cause poor circulation, chronic constipation, incontinence, weak muscles, weakened bone structure, pressure sores, increased agitation, loss of mobility, depressed appetite, increased threat of pneumonia, increased urinary infections, or death. Restraints also reduce the quality of life and, by their very nature, can cause withdrawal from surroundings, diminished social contact, depression, increased problems with sleep, and agitation.

If the nursing home you are considering is interested in restraint reduction, suggest that its director contact the National Citizens' Coalition for Nursing Home Reform (see Appendix C, "Community Resources") for materials that provide information on specific programs for reducing restraint use.

## Activities and Entertainment

One of the reasons you may have decided to place your loved one in a facility is so that he or she will have more opportunities to socialize with others. When you inspect facilities, find out what kinds of organized recreational activities are provided for residents. People with Alzheimer's disease are generally less agitated and require less medication and physical restraint in facilities that have programs, such as music, exercise, bingo, dancing, and games, rather than those in which residents watch television all day.

In many of the best facilities, residents are free to choose among scheduled activities that interest them—socializing with others, getting fresh air in the outdoor area, watching television in the lounge, or just spending quiet time in their rooms. In addition to in-house activities, some facilities schedule trips to various places in the community. This, of course, varies according to the abilities of the residents and, in the case of AD patients, the stage of the disease.

Does the staff make an effort to promote individualized activity and encourage the residents to take part in regular activities? People with Alzheimer's disease often don't do well in crowds of unfamiliar people, but some variety keeps them interested and helps prevent behavior problems.

## Food Service

Last, but not least, is the quality of the food in the facility. Check the menus, but also make sure you visit around a mealtime so you can look at or even taste the food. Does the food seem balanced and nutritious, or bland and institutional? Don't forget to check out the kitchen. Is it clean? Are dishes, pots, and pans clean? Are there bugs?

Will the person with AD have any choice regarding his or her food? If your loved one has special dietary needs, ask if they can be accommodated. Check to see if food is available only during mealtimes or if snacking is possible. Also, find out if the person with AD can choose whether to eat in the privacy of his or her room or with others in a dining room. And is assistance available if the patient needs to be fed?

Finally, don't ignore your overall gut feeling about the facility and the staff. If you take time to do your homework, you will find the right facility for your loved one. Once you have chosen a home—depending on how long the waiting list is—you can start getting ready for the move.

# 23

# *Moving In*

―――――――――――― ❧ ――――――――――――

You have made the decision to place your loved one with Alzheimer's in a facility, and you have done your homework and found a home that you feel confident will give him or her the best possible care. Now it's time to move your loved one, and you may be worried about the impact that moving will have on him. The actual move, however, may be more traumatic for you than for the Alzheimer's patient. You will be painfully aware of what's happening and may have feelings of guilt. You may also feel afraid, isolated, and sad, while your loved one with AD may not even be very conscious of the change.

If you have taken care of the person with Alzheimer's for years, his care has filled your time and engaged all of your emotional energy. Now, you will be moving the person and coming home to an empty house. You will be giving up your role as primary caregiver to the staff of the facility you have chosen. In this chapter, we'll not only address some practical suggestions for making the move easier for the person with Alzheimer's, we'll also focus on ways for you to cope with this very significant change in your life.

*One Caregiver's Journey*

"My mother continued to live in her senior residence for a number of years after her diagnosis. I hired a woman to stay with her five days a week and the other two days she went to an Adult Day Care center. In the evenings, she was all right in the structured environment that she was used to at the residence, but I finally had to move her because people complained about her incontinence—she had accidents and wouldn't wear diapers. I was worried about moving her because she had been in the senior residence for 10 years. I thought she would object or be upset, but when I moved her, she seemed to think she was in the same place."

## A Smooth Transition

Your goal should be to make the change as painless as possible for both you and the person with AD. Here are some things you should keep in mind.

### What to Bring

What will you need to bring to the new residence? A good rule of thumb is to bring as much as you can to help the new home seem familiar to the person with AD without cluttering the room. As you know, clutter causes confusion in people with Alzheimer's, and it might also cause problems for the staff. If you are able to bring a favorite chair or other furnishings that the person with AD is attached to, arrange to do so. At a minimum, be sure to bring any mementos that the person enjoys, such as special photographs, a plant, a radio, or a favorite pillow.

Personalize the room as much as you can by hanging artwork and photos on the wall. Having familiar objects in the room will give the room a more personal feeling and whether or not it helps the person with AD adjust, it will make the room more welcoming for you and other family members.

The staff will let you know the types of clothing and personal items that you should bring. Sometimes, depending on the size of the facility, you will need to mark the clothing with the person's name or initials to make sorting after laundering easier for the staff. Don't feel that you must remember everything the first day. You can always bring additional items the next time you visit.

## Spend Time at the Facility

For many reasons, it's important for you to stay involved and visit the patient regularly. It will help you adjust to the change. It will help the person with AD adjust and will give the person invaluable personal attention, affection, and an important sense of continuity. Seeing your familiar face may be a great comfort to the person with AD and help him or her make the transition into a home more easily.

Not the least of reasons for visiting often and in an unscheduled manner is to make sure that the home is maintaining the best care for the Alzheimer's patient. Close monitoring on your part will ensure that your loved one's care does not slip below the highest level possible.

## Build Relationships with the Staff

It's important to realize that you are not relinquishing the care of your loved one to strangers. Get to know the nurses and nurse's aides who work at the facility on the different shifts. Most of them are very good at what they do. It takes a strong, compassionate person to do this kind of work. One of the rewards of their work may be the appreciation of family members for their efforts. Be sure you are kind to them, see them as individuals, and be appreciative of their work.

## The Patient's Reaction

The first question that may come to you as you anticipate the move is what should you say to the person with AD about it? That depends on both you and the Alzheimer's patient. You may want to discuss your decision and tell the person about the home. You may feel that if you don't, you are deceiving him or her. In general, although some people decide to fudge

If a new doctor will be attending the patient in the nursing home, be sure all medical records are sent to him or her. Ask your old doctor to call the new doctor and discuss the case. Let the new doctor know that you expect to be consulted on care decisions and look forward to being helpful, since you have a wealth of information about the person. But be prepared—it takes time to work well with a new doctor.

—————— 🦋 ——————

Some people with Alzheimer's disease resist nursing home placement. Your loved one may accuse you of abandoning him or may plead with you to take him home. The more guilt you harbor about the placement, the more this is likely to upset you. You're not abandoning him, however. You've made tremendous sacrifices to care for him, and may, in fact, have put off the nursing home transition longer than you should have. All you're doing is what must be done.

the truth a little, it's better to either tell the truth or say nothing. If you mislead the person by saying you're "just going for a visit" you could end up upsetting the person more than you would if you told the truth.

If the Alzheimer's patient had talked with you about the eventuality of a nursing home early on, or if she still has enough cognitive function to know what's happening, you should definitely inform her about the move. Those who are in the more advanced stage of the disease may be incapable of understanding the transition. In those cases, it's better to just not say anything because it is unlikely that she will understand. The most important thing, whether you tell the person about the move before it happens or not, is that you reassure her at the time of the move. Let your loved one know that you will be visiting frequently and that you are not far away if she needs you.

It's very important for you to spend as much time as possible at the facility right after the move. Beware of a facility that pressures you to leave the patient alone for the first few weeks. This approach to the patient's adjustment will only further frighten a person with AD. It will also make you feel helpless, on top of the already difficult emotions you are feeling.

## Sometimes It's Traumatic

Depending on the individual, the adjustment to the new surroundings and routines may be difficult. As you know, Alzheimer's patients don't do well with change—and this is a big change. Confronted with unfamiliar faces in an unfamiliar place, the person with AD may feel abandoned, lost, or deceived even if you have discussed the move with him or her. He or she may be angry, suspicious, or agitated, or may appear withdrawn and depressed. It's not uncommon for a person with Alzheimer's—depending on the stage of the disease—to frantically search a new place for something familiar.

You can help by being there as much as possible until the person with AD begins to adjust to the new surroundings. People have different adjustment periods, so be patient; your loved one will adjust eventually. If the person with Alzheimer's says the facility is abusive or begs to return home with you, make sure that no abuse has, in fact, taken place. If it hasn't, simply offer as much understanding and reassurance as you can. Tell the person with AD that he or she is not well enough to be at home anymore.

## Sometimes It's Positive

Not every person with Alzheimer's has a difficult time adjusting to the move to a nursing home or other facility. Your loved one may respond very positively to the new surroundings, the structured routine, and the chance for interaction with other residents and staff. Some AD patients actually improve when they leave their home for a facility.

# Your Reaction

You have been through a lot in dealing with this disease, but you may find that one of the most difficult times for you yet is the period following placing the person with AD in a facility. When it is your spouse, you must go through a separation and some difficult emotional adjustments following the placement. When it is your parent, you may have some equally powerful reactions. We'll discuss the coping problems both of partners or spouses and adult children in the following sections, but first we'll cover some issues that affect all caregivers, regardless of the relationship to the person with AD.

## A Change, Not a Defeat

If you have been a full-time caregiver for the person with AD, you may have feelings of loss, loneliness, and emptiness after the move of your loved one to a facility. You may find yourself crying more than ever before—now that you have the time to really feel. You may also have feelings of guilt and concerns about whether or not you have made the right decision.

Your adjustment may be easier if you can see the transition to a nursing facility as a change and not a defeat. You may have strived to take care of the person with AD at home for many years. You may feel defeated that you now have to turn that job over to others.

Problems may occur because of neglect or actual abuse. If you notice bruises or a sudden increase in symptoms such as incontinence, dehydration, pressure sores, agitation, or depression, there may be actual abuse or neglect in the facility. When you suspect abuse, it is critical that you report it immediately. Make your report to the nursing home's administrator, an ombudsman, the local police, or the state agency that licenses and certifies nursing homes. Make your report in writing and keep trying until you get the assistance you need. For more information on abuse and neglect in nursing homes, contact the National Citizens' Coalition for Nursing Home Reform (see Appendix C, "Community Resources).

———— ✱ ————

It may take a little time for the staff and other patients to get used to the new AD patient. At the same time, staff members who are experienced with the disease know that it generally takes time for a person with Alzheimer's to adjust to new surroundings. You can help the staff by sharing parts of the person's history so they can get to know him better and individualize his care.

———— ✱ ————

You aren't giving up the care of your loved one when you place her in a facility—you're simply delegating to someone else to provide that care. You can still have an active role. Remember that you are paying for a service, so you have a right to see that it's being done properly and that your loved one is getting the care she deserves. If you have a complaint, talk it over with whoever is in charge and persevere until you get satisfaction.

Another way to look at it, however, is to be proud of what you have accomplished as a caregiver. Let yourself feel satisfied by how much you did, rather than focusing on what you can no longer do. Think about it—you took on a task for which you were never trained. It was probably something you wouldn't have willingly chosen in a million years, but you did it. You learned to do things you never imagined you'd have to do. You provided loving care and now you will continue to do so, but with the professional support of the facility. It's a change—a big one—but not a defeat. The person with AD will still get the best care possible.

## Express Your Feelings

This is a time when you may find yourself filled with fears, worries, and pent-up, long-unexpressed feelings. You may be worrying about the care your loved one is receiving or you may be fearful about your own future. It's important that you reach out and talk to friends and relatives or members of your Alzheimer's support group at this time. You have time now to have lunch or dinner with a friend. Tell him or her about your feelings. Just talking about how you are feeling will do a world of good.

In addition to the obvious fears or worries, you probably have a lot of feelings that have been building up inside of you during the years of caregiving. These feelings may be about the person with AD or about the loss of the person. They may be about the disease and the unfairness of life. Or you may have strong feelings about the lack of support from other family members while you took on the burden of caring for the Alzheimer's patient.

Now is the time to let your feelings come out and work through them. A lot of grief, sadness, and anger can build up as you care for a person with Alzheimer's. Even though you may have been aware of trying to express your feelings, you may simply not have had the space and time to really deal with them. Now that you are no longer providing around-the-clock care, these feelings may suddenly emerge and hit you quite hard.

Even though the person is still alive, you are going through a period of grieving. It's important that you seek out your family and friends, your support group, or members of the clergy for help. If for some reason you don't feel comfortable talking about all of your feelings with friends or relatives, don't try to ignore them or hold them in at this critical time. See a therapist or counselor. If you haven't found one at earlier points in your caregiving journey, find one now.

---

*One Caregiver's Journey*

"I realized by listening to others in my support group how hard it is for spouses to place their partners in a home. No one can tell them that it's time. They have to decide for themselves. I thought one woman in my group would never place her husband, no matter how hard we tried to convince her that it was what she needed to do. Finally, she realized that she couldn't handle his care alone. Now, as much as she loves him and misses him, she has admitted to us that she couldn't go back and take care of him again. She knows he is happy and content. And, she, too, is more content. Before, she was concerned that if something happened to her, there would be no one to take care of him. Now, she doesn't have to worry."

---

If you aren't ready and willing to relinquish your role as caregiver, you may find yourself developing anger, envy, and competition toward the facility's staff. After all, they get to see your loved one every day and you don't. Feeling protective of her, you may be overly critical of the staff. Many people have these kinds of feelings, but ultimately, they aren't productive and don't help your loved one. Talk to a counselor if you can't control these feelings.

---

## When It's Your Partner

When we marry or commit ourselves to sharing our lives with another person, we expect to be there for that person until the end. Most of us believe that if we love someone, it means that we will nurture and take care of him or her. Now you have turned over the job of nurturing and caring for your life partner to the professional staff who work in the facility. You may feel that you have abandoned and deserted your loved one and broken your promises by doing so. Despite your logical feelings that you did the right thing, these feelings of guilt can overwhelm you.

Now that you are separated from your loved one, you may feel lonely and, of course, need to adjust to a single life. But you may be feeling so guilty for not being able to take care of

---
🌿
---

People may tell you that now that the person with AD is in a facility, you are finally free. In truth, you may not feel free at all. You still think about her. You check on her regularly to make sure she is all right. You hope that you can go on with your life, but you are filled with fears and worries. It will take time to adjust, so don't be hard on yourself if you don't feel "free."

---

him or her anymore that you aren't focusing on your sadness and your need to take care of yourself. If you feel relief, if you do something enjoyable or have a nice day on your own with friends, you may feel guilty because he or she is not with you.

You need to remember something you may have forgotten along the way—you have a life of your own. You don't need to let yourself be held hostage by Alzheimer's disease. When you promised to be there "until death do you part" you didn't conceive of the possible death of your loved one's memory that this disease has brought into your relationship before his or her actual death. Instead of being upset that you are no longer doing it all, try to take comfort in knowing that your partner is being taken care of each day by people who are trained to give the best possible care.

## Deal with Your Overwhelming Loss

You may feel that, in placing your spouse or partner, you have lost your purpose in life. In a sense, you have. You will need time to find other ways to create meaning and purpose in your life. The most important thing you can do for yourself at this time, however, is to rest and give yourself time to adjust and deal with your loss. Before you become involved in making new plans, take some time to recover. You will have the strength you need to make plans and act on them later on.

You may also experience a wrenching loneliness that you have never felt before. You were slowly losing your connection with the person with AD intellectually and emotionally. Now you don't even have his or her physical presence with you anymore. You may feel that you have been given the worst that life has to offer—you aren't widowed or divorced, but your spouse is not really there in any real way either. Although you may feel depressed and hopeless, try to remember that you are in the grieving process (see Chapter 16, "How Do You Survive Stage 3?") and it will not last forever. And, with a degenerative disease like Alzheimer's, grieving takes place at many points along the way, not simply at the time of death.

## Don't Stay Isolated

You may have had to neglect friendships while you were in the throes of caregiving and during the time immediately after the placement of your loved one in the nursing home. It's important to take the time to repair those relationships now that you have the time.

You may not only have backed away from friends in the middle of all the crises that Alzheimer's disease brings, but also your friends may have stopped calling you. Perhaps being around the person with AD made some of them feel uncomfortable. If you don't want to lose them, forgive them and reach out to them again. Old friends, who have known you through many different stages of your life, can be a great comfort.

If you don't want to, or can't, repair all of your old relationships, then make new friends. Remember, you are not the person you were before your years as a caregiver. You had to become stronger. You had to learn new things and become increasingly independent. Now, you are learning how to go on with your life. It might be the right time to find new friends—friends who can help you along in the next part of your journey.

## Start to Build a Single Life

If you have been married for many years, you must now face a whole new kind of life. Little things like shopping and cooking for one person instead of two will seem difficult and may bring strong emotions. One way to handle the change is to create a new routine and schedule for yourself, planning things that you enjoy for some part of each day.

You will ultimately have to decide how to fill the void in your life, but don't try to do it immediately. At some point, you may want to resume your work or volunteer activities that you have given up while taking care of the person with AD. What your life will become after the person in your care has moved to a new home depends on many factors. The main thing is to accept that now you do have a life of your own and you have the right to live it as you please.

———— 🦋 ————

It's important that you don't feel bad about the sacrifices you made in your own life to take care of the person with AD. You can feel comfort from the memories you have and give yourself credit for the skills and character traits you built during your years of caregiving. As you go back into the world, remember that you are a stronger person for the experience.

## When It's Your Parent

You may have taken care of your parent with AD for many years. You may have sacrificed your career or your social life, or both. You may have put stress on your relationship with your family and spouse by taking on the responsibility for your parent. Now that you have placed your mother or father in a facility, it's time to start to rebuild your life. How do you do it?

In some ways, your adjustment may just be as hard as that of the spouse who has been married to the Alzheimer's patient for many years. The spouse was expected to take on the care of his or her partner, but you chose to take on the Herculean task out of love for your parent. Now, you have had to give up in some ways. You still have responsibilities to your parent, but not full-time ones. In order to rebuild your life, you have to deal with your emotions and accept the challenge of repairing relationships and reentering the world of work.

As you learn to adjust to your new life, you will still have a life with the person with AD. You will just need to learn how to continue to connect with the person even though you no longer live in the same home.

# 24

# *Make Your Visits Count*

❧

At first, your visits to the Alzheimer's patient at his or her new home will help you adjust to the new situation. If you were the primary caregiver, the job has been so consuming that despite your best efforts to maintain friendships and other activities, you're quite likely to feel lost for a while and not part of the world beyond Alzheimer's care. Visits can help you feel that you're still connected to the person with AD and still providing some care, even as you withdraw from day-to-day responsibilities.

After a while, however, as the Alzheimer's patient's remaining abilities fade and his or her life is focused less on you and more on the new home, you may feel that your visits are awkward. It may be difficult for you to figure out what to do during your visits. As the disease progresses, your loved one may finally no longer recognize you. At that point, you may feel that your visits are pointless.

Don't stop visiting the Alzheimer's patient—no matter how pointless it may seem to you. You can find ways to make your visits satisfying, and even people in the late stage of the disease seem to gain a sense of reassurance from the presence of family members. In this chapter, you'll learn tips for making your visits as meaningful as possible for both you and the person with AD.

As you continue to visit your loved one, you will learn how to best interact with him or her in the new environment. At first, you may expect to have all of his or her attention when you

---
❦
---

It's not a good idea for several family members to visit at the same time, since it may add to your loved one's confusion and cause him or her to be more agitated than normally. And, as when he or she was at home, smaller children and their normal high level of energy and playfulness might be too much for the AD patient to handle.

---

visit, but it may not work out that way. If he or she is involved in a group activity or is in an unreceptive mood, just go with the flow. Also, each visit may be different, so allow for surprises.

## Create a Regular Visiting Routine

If you took care of the Alzheimer's patient at home, you learned that regular routines are important to people with AD. The same is true of his or her schedule at a nursing home. Your visits should be regular and should fit into the routine of the home. If you are visiting from a distance and cannot visit regularly, call ahead and make sure that the staff prepares your loved one for your visit.

Even when your visits are regular, or you have asked the staff to prepare the person for the visit, your arrival may still come as a surprise to him or her. Your loved one may seem agitated or may walk away in the middle of the conversation. If that happens, just let your loved one take the lead. If it's not a good time for a visit, you might need to do something very simple, such as take a quiet walk together. The important thing is for you to be flexible. You may have something planned—an outing or activity that you are looking forward to—but if it isn't a good time for the person with AD, be willing to do something else.

## Creative Ways to Connect

Visiting a person with Alzheimer's disease in a nursing home is not always an easy experience. Things will seem very different than they were when the two of you were together at home. In the beginning, you will probably have many questions. You won't have your daily home routine to discuss, so what should you talk about? How do you visit with him or her in front of all these other people? What should you do when other residents seek your attention?

Unlike at home, where the purpose of much of your interaction was to handle the routine and activities of daily life, in the nursing home, the staff takes care of most of that. Your visits will have different goals—to connect with the person, to share a moment, and to have a pleasant experience together.

To accomplish these goals, you have to be flexible and see what works. The following section provides some ideas that have worked for others, but also let what you know about the person with AD guide you. Remember that it's all right to have a visit with little or no conversation. Simply sitting together holding hands can be enjoyable for the person with AD.

Finally, remember that as the disease progresses, the person will be changing. Let the staff guide you when he seems to reject activities that were once enjoyable to him.

## One Caregiver's Journey

"My brother, who lived in the East, used to come out to visit every year, and I would take him over to visit our mother. I think she usually recognized him, but I'm not sure. It's typical of all adult children to want to see our parents more together, in better shape, but Alzheimer's disease is so humiliating. By the time my mother was in the facility, she rarely wore her own clothes. The staff couldn't take the time to separate everyone's clothes, and often the patients themselves would go around and take clothes out of the other residents' drawers and closets. They would take anything that was loose. I had brought over two very nice outfits for my mother not long before one of my brother's visits. I said to the owner, 'Please, when I bring my brother over tomorrow, I want to have my mother in one of these two outfits.' I knew my mother didn't care by that time, but it was for the family. So she looked really good that day, and I was pleased that my brother saw her that way."

## Bring a Favorite Food

The way to your Alzheimer's patient's heart—if he or she is not in the late stage of the disease—may still be through his or her stomach. Rather than expecting to sit and talk throughout your visit, bring in some of the person's favorite foods to share. Your loved one might appreciate a special main dish or dessert. The food might also serve as a topic for discussion. If

—————— ❧ ——————

When talking with someone who has Alzheimer's disease, the content of the conversation is much less important than how the affected person feels about the conversation. You don't have to correct your loved one if he or she says something you know is incorrect. If he or she confuses the year or calls you by the wrong name, it's not important. Ask general questions, rather than focusing on details that he or she is likely to have forgotten already.

—————————————

it's a small facility or if you have the use of the kitchen and you and the person with AD like to cook, you might be able to even prepare a favorite treat together.

## Decorate the Patient's Room for Holidays

The community rooms of the facility may be filled with holiday decorations, but your loved one's room may look drab in comparison. You might be able to brighten his or her spirits by bringing in some personal holiday decorations for him or her. Be careful, however, that nothing you bring in is dangerous. If you have questions, the staff can guide you.

If the person with AD has a birthday, you can bring in banners to let everyone in the facility know about it. You can bring greeting cards from long distance relatives and, of course, presents. Make a celebration out of not just birthdays, but other holidays. The person with AD will probably delight in seeing you decorate and organize the celebration. He or she may just want to watch or may participate along with you.

## Personal Grooming for Fun and Relaxation

Other activities that you can share with the Alzheimer's patient are various personal grooming activities. For example, you can give the person a manicure or a pedicure. Or you might be able to provide a shave, a shampoo, a new hairdo, or some sort of beauty treatment. Even simply brushing or combing the person's hair can be a nice way to spend time together.

Perhaps the person always enjoyed having her shoulders rubbed. If so, you can pamper her with a little shoulder, hand, neck, or foot massage using essential oils and fragrances. Even something simple like bringing a nice-smelling hand lotion, perfume, or after-shave lotion can bring pleasure to the person with AD and thus enhance your visit.

## Bring Scrapbooks and Old Pictures

As Alzheimer's disease progresses, as you know, those who are affected are able to remember fewer events that happened in recent years, months, or days. Most of what they are able to remember happened many years ago and is stored in their long-term memory. When you visit, it's often better to draw upon these past events than to talk about what happened over the weekend or that morning. Favorite anecdotes from the past can be told over and over and continue to delight the person with AD.

It also can be fun to bring old family pictures or scrapbooks for you and the person with AD to look at. You may have wondered why you took so many pictures in the past. Now you have a use for them. Organizing pictures, old clippings, old greeting cards, letters, or other mementos into scrapbooks can be an activity that you and the person with AD can spend time on during many visits. Once the scrapbooks or photo albums are made, you can use them to either stimulate a conversation about past events or just to look at over and over.

Photos or slides, rather than videos or films, are generally better for people with Alzheimer's because the fast movement in the videos may be hard for the person to process. You can bring videotapes of family visits when family members live far away, but remember to shoot them without a lot of background noise and camera movements.

If the person's reading skills have deteriorated, you can make audiotapes of a favorite author's short stories or a favorite poet. Music may also stimulate memories and conversations and provide hours of enjoyment. Bring your loved one a portable cassette player and headphones so she can enjoy the music after you leave.

## Outings

What about taking the person with AD out for a meal, to a park, the zoo, the beach, an art exhibition, or a museum? Sometimes, outings can be very successful, particularly when the surroundings aren't loud, noisy, or confusing. A walk in a quiet park might be extremely rewarding, but a visit to a busy, noisy restaurant—even one with good food—might prove disastrous.

When you are visiting a nursing home, other residents will often try to join in your conversation or activities. Don't be disturbed by it. After several visits, having extra people around will probably seem normal, and it may help the visit to go more smoothly. If you would like to have privacy for some reason, ask the staff for a room where you can meet with your loved one without any distractions.

—————— 🦋 ——————

Most activities are meaningful for the Alzheimer's patient because of the relationship he or she shares with you. As the disease progresses, you might want to rely more on familiar outings that you know the person with AD enjoys. A break in the routine, though refreshing for you, may produce stress and discomfort for the person with AD. Familiarity, not variety, is the Alzheimer's patient's spice of life.

Here are some guidelines for choosing outings:

- Go to places at times when there are fewer people so as not to over-stimulate the person. For example, an early dinner at a restaurant might be better than at a busy time.
- Limit the time spent on one activity to less than a few hours. Activities that last longer are often too difficult for the person with AD.
- Plan activities that allow you to be flexible, and change plans if necessary.
- Plan activities that don't require much concentration, but still hold the person's attention—such as a visit to a pet store, the zoo, or a flower shop.
- Don't expect the AD patient to do more than he or she wants to do or seems capable of doing.
- Plan simple activities that are not demanding, such as a walk in the park, getting an ice-cream cone, or stopping at the local nursery.
- Be creative and try things that might be out of the ordinary such as going to a garage sale or visiting a history or science museum.
- Plan activities that include sensory experiences, such as smelling the aroma of freshly baked bread or petting a puppy.
- Find quiet places, such as an outing to the library or a stroll through an arboretum or gardens.

In the days and weeks after you have placed the Alzheimer's patient in the new facility, she may ask you to take her "home." If you do so and make that the outing for the day, she may want to leave soon after you arrive. The word "home" may now mean the nursing home or it may have some other meaning in her mind.

## Visits During Scheduled Activities

It's best for you to become part of the patient's routine at the facility, rather than having your visits disrupt them. Since activities are scheduled regularly, you might want to plan your visit while certain activities are taking place. Attending a party, a craft session, or a game at the facility can help make the time more pleasant. Some days you may simply want to observe the activity, and sometimes you may want to join in with the group. Check with the staff to see which activities would be most suitable for you to attend with your loved one.

*One Caregiver's Journey*

"After I placed my mother in a facility, she took a liking to a man in a wheelchair who had had a stroke. This is a common thing that happens. My mother was always talking to this man, but his stroke had left him unable to speak. She had always done all the talking when my father was alive, too. One day I said to her, 'Do you want to go for a walk, Mother?' She said, 'Just a minute, I'll ask your father if he wants to go.' I said to her, 'Mother, he may be your husband, but he is not my father.' She still liked the men to the end and they liked her. Often, if there is a healthy spouse involved in a situation like this one, they get jealous. This man was married, but his wife didn't seem to mind. I was there one time and I said to her, 'My mother seems to like your husband. I hope you don't mind.' She said, 'Listen, anything that will give them pleasure at this point ...' That was nice, but it isn't the usual attitude."

## Positive Feedback

If you visit the person often, you will certainly experience a time when he or she seems in particularly good spirits or when his or her memory seems much better than usual. Be sure to praise the patient when that happens, but don't expect that it means he or she is getting better. As we discussed in earlier chapters on the stages of the disease, there are days when things are better and days when they are worse, but Alzheimer's is relentless—it won't go away.

Don't limit your praise and positive feedback to those times when the patient is particularly lucid. Being kind and positive with the person with AD will make your visits more enjoyable both for him and for you. Positive feedback from you will

---🦋---

The feelings you share during a visit are more important than the content of your conversation. The person may no longer know who you are, but will know that she is in the presence of someone who cares about her. Sometimes the Alzheimer's patient will no longer recognize you and will hold hands with another resident. Chances are she thinks she is with you. You don't need to set the record straight. Just continue to show your love for her.

---

reassure him and make him feel loved. Feeling the love of others is important for all of us and that is true of Alzheimer's patients as well, even in the late stages of the disease.

## How to Handle an Upsetting Visit

Sometimes a visit with the Alzheimer's patient, despite your best efforts, will be an utter failure. He or she may be agitated or seem totally unreachable the entire time you are there. You had hoped for a connection, but it was impossible. Or, it may be the first time that you really feel the person with AD doesn't recognize you at all. He may think you are someone else. During the visit, you didn't correct or argue with him and you tried not to be upset in his presence. Now, however, it really hurts. Perhaps the person had a catastrophic outburst or seemed angry with you. Perhaps he said things in anger that made you feel really bad.

In any of these instances, you may leave the facility feeling sad and upset. Unfortunately, nothing can really prevent unsuccessful moments or painful visits. It is the nature of the disease. Watching your loved one drift away is heart-rending and deeply disappointing. But for your health and for the well-being of your loved one, you should try to find ways of coping with the emotions that the unhappy visit brings.

First, it's important that you don't deny your feelings, try to shrug them off, or keep them bottled up inside. Talk with friends, family, members of your support group, or a professional counselor. Let yourself receive the support and insight that others can give you at this time when you are upset. Also, try to focus on the good times and the good memories of your life with your loved one. You have wonderful shared experiences that are still part of your life together. They shouldn't be erased because your loved one has Alzheimer's. Remember that it is the disease that is causing the person's behavior—it's not about you at all.

Try to see humor in the situation—if you can find any. Also try to see that it's not really logical to expect that someone who has a disease that is destroying his or her entire memory should remember you. Of course, emotions aren't logical, but as time goes by, you will develop more tolerance and acceptance of what the disease is doing to your loved one.

Be sure to visit again soon after a bad visit. Each visit is different, and both you and your loved one are likely to be in a different mood the next time you see one another. Don't deny yourself a pleasurable visit because of the experience of a painful one. Focus on the positive aspects of the situation instead of the person's deterioration.

## Keep in Touch with the Staff

As time goes by, get to know the staff and make a habit of sharing things with them about the person with AD. Tell them about activities that he or she enjoyed with you or about ones that he or she didn't like. See if staff members have ideas for new activities.

If you were the primary caregiver for a person with Alzheimer's, you know how difficult it is to take care of someone with the disease. So, have empathy for the staff members of a nursing home or other facility who have a number of people with AD to care for. Give them your respect and support. If you're appreciative of them and develop a rapport with them, they are likely to take a more personal interest in your loved one. You can support the staff members—particularly those who seem to really care about their jobs—by encouraging them to think creatively about new ways to meet residents' needs. Show them that you are a partner, not an adversary, and it will be good for the staff, for the person with AD, and for you.

You may not be able to visit as often as you want to, but you can still check up on your loved one by phone. When you do so, always ask specific questions about his or her condition, rather than general ones. For example, instead of "How's my mother?" ask: "What portion of her dinner did she eat? Did she take part in the group activities today?" Be specific and you will receive more accurate information.

# 25

# *The Present: Caring for Yourself Through It All*

Caregiving, as you know, is a time-consuming job. Approximately 20 percent of caregivers have to quit their jobs and 40 percent have to reduce their work hours in order to provide care for an Alzheimer's patient. And not only is being a caregiver for an affected person time-consuming, it is also a very stressful job.

Stress has been shown to either cause or exacerbate 70 to 90 percent of all medical conditions, including tension and migraine headaches, high blood pressure, asthma, nervous stomach, bowel problems, and chronic lower back pain. Stress also increases a person's susceptibility to far more serious conditions, such as heart disease, stroke, and cancer. Stress has also been tied to numerous psychological problems, such as anxiety, depression, phobias, drug and alcohol abuse, and insomnia.

How do you deal with the stress of caregiving without getting sick yourself? When you go out for a jog or a walk, you have to decide which path you should take. You can walk along the side of a busy street, breathe in the toxic automobile fumes, and listen to the roar of engines, screeching tires, and honking horns. Or you can find a more serene place to walk that is away from the noisy traffic—on a side street past homes with flower beds or in a park with trees and children playing. In much the same way, you have a choice of the kind of path to take on your journey as a caregiver. Will you just accept the inevitable stress of the situation, or will you take steps to make the journey a little easier? In this chapter, you'll get to look at some signposts that may lead you to the more peaceful road to take.

In previous chapters, we've discussed a number of things you should do to care for yourself during specific stages of Alzheimer's disease. This chapter both reviews some of those suggestions and offers additional ideas and techniques for reducing stress and staying healthy.

### One Caregiver's Journey

"It was a long, trying experience taking care of my mother after she developed Alzheimer's, but I survived by taking care of myself. I think it's crucial to get help and take care of yourself so that you will be better able to take care of the person in your life. You are important, too. Just because she's sick, she's not more important than you. And you *can* do both. It's not an either-or situation. You can take very good care of her and also take good care of yourself."

## Empathy for You

By now, you should have a pretty good understanding of the world in which the person with Alzheimer's lives. You have learned how the brain damage from the disease affects his or her behavior, and that understanding has given you empathy for his or her limitations, feelings, and motives for various behaviors.

You have come to understand that it's futile to try to keep the person with AD in your world. You realize that it isn't fair to expect someone with Alzheimer's to do things he or she used to do when, given the brain damage that has occurred, it's impossible for him or her to function in the same way. You have learned not to insist on behavior that isn't possible anymore.

The empathy you developed for the person with AD helps you in your role as a caregiver because it allows you to see life—as much as you can—as the person with AD sees it. You try to let the Alzheimer's patient live in his or her world and accept that you no longer share the same reality.

To be a successful caregiver, however, you also need to develop empathy for yourself. You need to be able to give yourself the same understanding and sympathy that you have learned to give to the Alzheimer's patient. Take time to stand back and look at yourself from a distance—not in a critical way, but with empathy. Make a list of your strengths and weaknesses. From them, learn to appreciate yourself for what you can do; and don't expect the impossible of yourself, just as you wouldn't of the person with AD.

## Your Limits and Limitations

It's very important for you to know what your limits are, so you don't burn yourself out. You also need to be aware of your limitations or weaknesses, so you don't expect more from yourself than you can effectively give. We all have talents—skills that we perform better than we do other things. You may be great in the kitchen—you can whip up something delicious quickly—but you may get upset or be impatient with the person with AD when he or she needs a bath. With that knowledge of yourself, why not hire someone who can help the Alzheimer's patient with his or her baths and personal hygiene? If you can't afford it, ask other relatives to chip in for the cost of a part-time home health aide.

Be honest in your assessment of your limits and limitations as a caregiver, so that you can set realistic goals. If you know your limits, you can ask family members or friends to help or you can find out if there are community services available to fill those voids. If you recognize what you can and cannot do, define your priorities, and act accordingly, you will be much better off than if you try to do it all yourself and soon find that you are more and more stressed out because you can't. There is no shame in not being able to do it all. If you know and accept your limits, you will also be better able to plan for the next stages of the AD patient's care.

## Staying in Balance

You may feel that you are taking care of yourself, but perhaps you are not looking at your situation in an objective way. How can you evaluate yourself so that you really know whether or not you are undervaluing your needs in relation to those of the person with Alzheimer's? When is caregiving out of balance?

First, what are the extremes of caregiving? On one hand, a caregiver may not provide enough care for the Alzheimer's patient. He or she may abandon, neglect, or even abuse the person with AD. Unfortunately, as horrible as this seems, it does happen. Not only are there cases of actual physical neglect in which an affected person is exposed to life-threatening situations, but some caregivers may also emotionally neglect an Alzheimer's patient. A caregiver can refuse to give the person affection, display coldness, anger, detachment, or no genuine concern, providing for only the minimal physical needs of the person with AD.

On the other extreme is the caregiver who is over-involved with caring for the person with Alzheimer's to the point of ignoring his or her own needs. This type of caregiver frantically attempts to provide for every possible need of the patient. The person with AD is not allowed any independence, and the caregiver entirely abandons his or her own needs to provide for the needs of the person with Alzheimer's. Do you know Alzheimer's caregivers who are like that? Do you have a tendency to be over-involved?

How do you find a path between those two extremes, and what does that path look like? You of course need to be concerned with both the emotional and physical well-being of the person you are caring for. You have to develop empathy for the Alzheimer's patient so you can understand his or her limits and problems. But at the same time, you have to find time to care for yourself. When you make a schedule of daily activities and routines for the Alzheimer's patient, is there time on the schedule each day for you to go to your special place to be alone? Is there time for a relaxing activity for you? If not, you may be focusing too much attention on the Alzheimer's patient and not enough on yourself.

The key is to find a balance between under-care and over-care, and to balance your own needs with those of the Alzheimer's patient. Neither of the two extremes is healthy—for you or for the person with AD. At the same time that you show your respect and love for the Alzheimer's patient, you must also respect and value your own needs as an individual and as a caregiver.

## Signs of Stress

How do you know if you are becoming overly stressed or near burnout? Just as the Alzheimer's Association developed the very comprehensive and informative "Warning Signs of Alzheimer's Disease" covered in Chapter 2, "When to Worry: The Ten Warning Signs of Alzheimer's," it has also published a list of signs of impending caregiver stress. We'll summarize those signs here, but you also might want to request a copy of the Association's free brochure, "Caregiver Stress: Signs to Watch for ... Steps to Take" and keep it by your bedside. Learning about Alzheimer's disease has helped you cope with taking care of the person with AD and learning about your own potential condition—caregiver stress or burnout—will help you prevent and cope with it.

What are the signs of caregiver stress? Stress may manifest differently in different people. The following are some common warning signs of caregiver stress.

- Denial about the person with Alzheimer's disease—a caregiver may think the AD patient might get better
- Frequent anger or irritability—constantly snapping at the person with AD or others, even over little things
- Sleep problems, such as exhaustion, insomnia, or constant fatigue or pressure—may be unable to fall asleep for hours or sleep restlessly all night long
- Difficulty concentrating
- Social withdrawal, anxiety, or depression—refusing to go out at all, claiming the person with AD needs him or her
- Constant worry
- Lack of motivation to even get out of bed

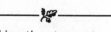

Taking time to meet your needs has a tremendous payoff in terms of your ability to deal with emotional stress. To successfully use any activity for stress reduction or simply enjoyment, however, you must plan and set up a specific time when it can be done. The activity won't happen by just saying that you should do it. You must make a definite plan and follow through.

—————— ❧ ——————

Do you seldom laugh anymore? Do you find yourself yelling, screaming, or having crying fits or rages frequently? Do you withhold affection or even withhold food, baths, dressing changes, or other assistance from the affected person? Are you constantly blaming him or her for your being in this situation? Do you withhold expenditures for needed goods or services because it's wasting money? If any of these behaviors occur, you need to take time off immediately and get psychological help.

———————————————

- Chronic health problems—which can be caused or exacerbated by stress

If you are regularly experiencing any of these signs, it's extremely important that you learn and use various techniques for stress reduction that we'll cover later in this chapter, that you get emotional support and also get help so you can get away for extended periods. If you don't take steps to decrease your stress level, both for your own well-being and for that of the person with AD, it's time to stop being a caregiver.

# The Physical Part of Staying Healthy

Caring for yourself has to start with your body. Chances are that, despite all the warnings in previous chapters, you still don't give your body enough sleep, enough nutritious food, or enough exercise. You might also skip regular medical checkups and maybe even abuse your body by smoking cigarettes or drinking too much alcohol. You may have been able to get away with those bad habits in your old life. In your life as a caregiver for an Alzheimer's patient, however, you aren't going to make it for the long haul unless you take care of yourself while you are caring for the person with AD.

## Sleep and Relaxation

Sleep refreshes you and enables you to function throughout the day. If the person with Alzheimer's is restless at night and disturbs your sleep and nothing you do seems to alleviate the problem, you may have to obtain outside help in the evenings so you can get a good night's sleep. If you are unable to sleep because of tension, try meditation or relaxation exercises. (See more on these techniques later in this chapter.) If nothing works and you experience continued sleep disturbances, it may be a sign of depression, and you should see a doctor or therapist.

Along with getting enough sleep, you need to be sure that you also take time to relax. Plan some type of leisure or relaxing activity each day and you will be amazed at how it will help.

You'll feel better and be better able to cope with your situation. Take time to read a book, telephone a friend, or watch a favorite television show or video. Even an hour a day will help alleviate your stress and lift the burden of your caregiving responsibilities.

## Diet

Good food is the fuel that your body needs to function. By now, you know that you need to eat three simple, nutritious, well-balanced meals a day to be able to keep up your strength and stay healthy under the stress of your duties as a caregiver. If you skip meals, eat poorly or drink lots of caffeine, your body will rebel by getting sick. When you are shopping for groceries and you feel like treating yourself to your favorite soda or candy bar, remember that juice, fruit, or a healthy snack like yogurt or a granola bar will be a lot better in the long run. You may even develop a taste for some of the healthy snacks that are available.

## Exercise

We've talked about exercise before and must mention it again here because it really is extremely important to your well-being, both physically and psychologically. Doing some sort of physical exercise every day—or at least three or four times a week—can relax you, boost your immune system, keep your muscles from tightening, and prevent chronic back pain and headaches. Stretching, walking, jogging, swimming, bicycling, working out at a gym, or any exercise you enjoy will give you an overall feeling of relaxation and just make you feel good.

If you haven't exercised much in your life, it may be hard to get into a routine, but once you do you will be amazed at the benefits you'll feel after only a few weeks. Some of your stress will evaporate and you'll definitely feel calmer and more relaxed. If you don't know what to do and how to begin, consult your doctor before starting an exercise routine. He or she can help design a program that fits your individual needs.

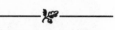

Even though you may feel like a stiff drink would help you relax after a hard day, in fact, alcohol has the opposite effect on the body. If you drink alcohol before going to bed, it may help you fall asleep, but you are likely to awaken in the middle of the night and not be able to get back to sleep. Avoid alcohol and never have more than two or three ounces when you do drink it.

How do you find time to eat right, exercise, and go in for check-ups, much less relax, when you don't even know how to find the time to care for the Alzheimer's patient and take care of your household? You may have to break some old habits. Let the dust build up. Don't scrub the floor as often. Or get some help. However you do it, your own health is a top priority and you must take time to stay healthy.

## Regular Medical Care

You may not feel that you need to make an appointment with your doctor for a regular checkup—you're too busy and you don't think there is anything wrong with you. Of course you're too busy and, hopefully, there isn't anything wrong with you, but during your time as a full-time caregiver, you need regular medical care more than ever. The stress you are under may cause minor problems that can turn into serious conditions if not treated. Doctors can detect developing problems through blood tests and other tests that are part of a routine examination.

# The Mental and Spiritual Parts of Staying Healthy

Taking care of your body is an essential part of relieving the stress of being a caregiver, but you also need to do things to take care of your mind and your spirit. We now know that the mind has an extraordinary ability to influence the body. In Chapter 9, "How Do You Survive Stage 1?" we discussed the importance of laughter and humor, and also suggested that you keep a journal. Laughing and writing in a journal, however, are only two popular ways to reduce stress. There are many other methods for reducing tension, and we'll go over some of them in the following sections. The important thing is to find the particular stress-reducer or combination of stress-reducing techniques that work best for you.

The first step, of course, is to admit to yourself that your stress or tension won't simply go away unless you find ways to reduce it.

## Meditation

Meditation is an ancient technique used in many cultures for both relaxation and enlightenment. In meditation practice, you learn to shut off your normal, thinking mind by focusing on something constant, such as your breathing or the flame of a candle. When your distracting thoughts start to fade, your mind is then free to feel and to contemplate. Because it can help you get in touch with your feelings, meditation may aid you in releasing pent-up feelings of sadness, grief, or anger. Meditation is often very successful in putting fears, anxieties, and disappointments in perspective and thus reducing stress.

There are many meditation techniques and schools for learning meditation. You can buy books on meditation, go onto the Internet to check out Web sites about meditation, or—and this is perhaps best—find a class at a local alternative healing or meditation center. Try to find a meditation instructor who uses meditation as a means of stress-reduction, healing, and increasing one's ability to feel.

Meditation isn't easy for everyone, and at first the results might be very subtle. If you continue to meditate regularly, however, your ability to shut down your busy, thinking mind will increase. Eventually, you will become so proficient that you can turn off your thinking mind at will and feel whatever is there.

No matter what type of meditation you learn, remember that the goal is to discover your inner self and increase your ability to feel. Don't get sidetracked by focusing on the technique. And when looking for a meditation instructor, follow your intuition. Do you feel comfortable around the person? Do you feel accepted by him or her? If not, look elsewhere. Your goal at this stressful time in your life is to relax, not to please a demanding instructor or become a monk.

## Relaxation Exercises

Meditation is a kind of relaxation exercise, but there are also even simpler relaxation techniques that you can use. When your physical body is relaxed, you don't need to be in such conscious control of your mind, and you can give it the freedom to daydream and use guided imagery or visualization techniques, which we'll discuss in the following sections.

To begin a simple relaxation exercise, loosen your clothing, take off your shoes, and sit comfortably in a quiet place where you won't be disturbed for a few minutes. You might want to play soft music or a CD with the sounds of waves or rain or something soothing to you. Close your eyes and take in a few

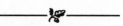

Meditation is a spiritual practice, not a religious practice. People may meditate whether they are atheists, Jewish, Christian, Buddhist, Moslem, Hindu, or Ba'hai. Different people benefit from different kinds of meditation, and you might want to find a kind of meditation that's consistent with your religious beliefs or lack of them. There are types of meditation that are common to each major religion, and some forms of meditation are compatible with all beliefs.

deep breaths. Then, picture yourself descending an imaginary staircase. With each step, notice that you feel more and more relaxed. You can also focus on each part of your body and feel it gradually become more relaxed. When your body feels relaxed, begin to imagine a favorite scene. It could be a beach, a deep green forest, or a particularly enjoyable moment with friends or family. Become totally immersed in the scene. Smell the smells. See the sights it offers. Hear the sounds. See yourself in that scene, relaxed and happy. At the end of your session, take a few more deep breaths and picture yourself climbing the imaginary staircase. Gradually become aware of your surroundings, open your eyes, stretch, and go on with your day.

Though there are infinite variations, this is all there is to a relaxation exercise. You can buy audiotapes or CDs or read books with more sophisticated ideas. You can play a tape that will lead you into your scene in a step-by-step manner. Then, once you are relaxed and comfortable in your favorite scene, you can use a specific guided imagery or visualization to gradually direct your mind toward an emotional issue or physical condition you're concerned about.

## Guided Imagery or Visualization

Guided imagery or visualization involves replacing negative images with positive ones. We have images and thoughts running through our minds all day, and many of them are harmful, negative images and worries. A steady dose of worries will increase stress and make the likelihood of illness greater. During guided imagery, you visualize a goal you want to achieve—such as getting rid of your tension headaches—and then imagine yourself going through the process of achieving it.

Imagery is as simple as a relaxation exercise. The first step, in fact, is to use a relaxation exercise to go to your favorite place in your mind. Once you are there, use an image that has some meaning to you or some connection to the problem you want to deal with. For example, some people actually personify their condition and try to reason with it. For tension headaches, you might imagine a gremlin tightening a vice across your head and causing it to ache. Ask the gremlin why he's there and what you can do to make him loosen his grip. The gremlin's answer might surprise you—maybe he'll chastise you for not getting enough sleep, exercise, or nutritious food. Negotiate an agreement with him—you'll get some sleep and he'll go away. Amazingly enough, there's a good chance that your headaches will start to subside.

There are books and tapes on guided imagery and visualization, and you can use images suggested by experts or make up your own. When you practice a visualization, try to let the image become more vivid and focused, but don't worry if it seems to fade in and out. If several images come to mind, choose one and stick with it for that session. If no images come to mind, think about how you feel at the moment. Are you angry or frustrated? What color is your anger? Try to make the color fill your visual field. Next, try concentrating on the color you have associated with the negative emotion and then mentally replace it with a soothing color that you associate with relaxation. For example, imagine the color red as your anger or stress and see it change to a peaceful, serene sky blue. Each time you do a visualization exercise, imagine that your ailment or your stress is completely gone at the end of the session.

Once you learn visualization techniques, you can use them every day. People often visualize in bed in the morning or at night before falling asleep. It's a good idea to practice imagery for 15 to 20 minutes a day initially to ensure that you're learning to do it properly. As you become more skilled and comfortable with the technique, you'll be able to do it for a few minutes at different times throughout the day. Depending on how stressed you are, you might see results right away, or it might take several weeks of using the technique to notice the change.

Many studies have shown imagery to be very effective in the treatment of stress and other conditions. In one study, researchers found that people with cancer who used imagery while receiving chemotherapy felt more relaxed, better prepared for their treatment, and more positive about their care than those who didn't use the technique. Another study demonstrated that patients suffering from severe depression were helped by imagining scenes in which they were praised by people they admired—a clear boost to their self-esteem. In still another study, researchers asked 19 men and women who had chronic bronchitis and emphysema, ages 56 to 75, to rate their levels of anxiety, depression, fatigue, and discomfort before and after they began using imagery. The researchers concluded that imagery significantly improved the overall quality of these people's lives. Imagery works, so it's worth trying!

## Breathing Exercises

Since childhood, when you've been upset, you may have been told to take a deep breath and calm down. Well, that's one of those clichés that is actually filled with quite a bit of wisdom. Not just any kind of breathing, but deep breathing from your diaphragm can help you release stress. Check yourself in the mirror when you take a deep breath. Does your chest expand and your stomach go in? If so, you are probably not breathing deeply from your diaphragm. To do so, you need to inhale so that your stomach sticks out instead of in.

If you have ever noticed a baby's abdomen rise and fall with each breath, you have seen proper deep breathing. Most adults tend to fill only the upper chest when they breathe and don't receive the benefit of the increased oxygen intake of a deep breath. A real deep breath helps to relieve tension and improve mental alertness.

Here's a simple deep breathing exercise for stress: Sit up straight in a chair, place one hand on your abdomen and breathe in deeply through your nose counting to ten. Hold the breath for a count of five, then release slowly through your mouth for a count of ten. While holding your breath, focus on your abdomen. Is it extended as far as you can comfortably extend it? Start with five of these exercises, but even two will help relieve stress.

Deep breathing exercises have been used for centuries as a way of relaxing the body. If you are uncertain that you are breathing properly, try taking a yoga, meditation, or voice class that focuses on how to breathe deeply. Once you learn how to breathe so that you actually fill your lungs to capacity, you can do a few regular, rhythmic, deep breaths whenever you want to. It's a fast, easy way to reduce stress and face the challenges of your day feeling calmer.

## Get a Massage

Until now, we've been focusing on things you can do yourself to relieve your stress and tension. Sometimes, however, it's good to treat yourself to a massage. Being touched by a skilled massage therapist is a wonderful way to not only relax your muscles, but also to reduce stress. Massage works by increasing the blood circulation and bringing more oxygen to sore, stiff muscles, which in turn helps to eliminate toxins that have accumulated in strained or overworked muscles. By relaxing your muscles and your body, massage can help alleviate conditions such as headaches, backaches, insomnia, and anxiety.

If you aren't familiar with massage, some of the types of massage available are:

- **Swedish.** Developed by a Swedish doctor, this is the most common type of massage in the U.S. It focuses on relaxation and is a fairly gentle, light-touch massage.
- **Deep-Tissue.** This type of massage focuses on loosening tight muscles. It is a harder massage and can hurt those who aren't used to it.
- **Acupressure.** This technique focuses on blocked areas. It's often helpful in improving the immune system and general well-being.
- **Shiatsu.** A Japanese massage technique similar to acupressure that uses strong, rhythmic pressure to release blocked energy.
- **Reflexology.** A very relaxing massage technique that works on the feet or hands.

Before making an appointment for a massage, get your questions answered so you won't be upset afterward and destroy the goal of the massage. Find out if the massage is done with or without clothes. How much does it cost? How long is the appointment? Can you have it done in your house? Are scented oils used? Is it a gentle massage or is it deeper?

During a massage, don't be afraid to ask to have the pressure changed if it is too light or too hard. Tell the massage therapist where you hurt so he or she can focus on where you need it most. And make sure you are comfortable. If you are too warm or too cold, say something.

To get the most out of your massage, rest, take a short walk, or sit quietly afterward to allow your body to adjust to its new, relaxed state. Also, drink lots of water. This helps the body flush out the toxins that were released from your muscles during the massage. After some massages, a warm bath can be nice, but if your massage therapist used aromatic oils you may not want to wash them off.

## Be Good to Yourself

Make sure you give yourself a daily or a weekly reward for your hard work as a caregiver. Make a list of the kinds of things that are rewards for you. Time for one of the activities that you enjoy may be one way to reward yourself, but there are other ways also. Maybe a special—and hopefully healthy—treat after dinner would be a way of rewarding yourself. Maybe your reward is a new item of clothing. Maybe it's the chance to watch your favorite television show. Maybe it's taking a few minutes to listen to your favorite music. Discover the small things in life that delight you and make you feel rewarded. Maybe it's a short chat with a close friend or relative. We are all different, and different activities engender in each of us different feelings. Working in the garden may simply be a chore for one person, but for you it may be a wonderful reward.

One of the most painful things you may have lost, as your loved one's disease has progressed, is the positive feedback he or she used to give you. The person with AD might have regularly complimented you on your appearance or expressed his or her pride in your accomplishments, but now, because of the disease, he or she rarely talks about you—except possibly to complain.

Now, you have to boost your self-esteem yourself. Take a minute to think about all that you have accomplished and all that you have learned as a caregiver. You have learned some very profound and character-building lessons on this journey, and you deserve to give yourself credit and accolades. Be proud of yourself—of your strength, your courage in facing the disease, your hard work, and your good humor through it all.

## One Caregiver's Journey

"I grew into the experience of being a caregiver for an Alzheimer patient and so will you. My success in handling the early problems built my confidence and I felt I could handle those that came toward the end. I learned to see my role in a positive way and not as drudgery or obligation. It took imagination, but I eventually worked out my own ways of not only doing the tasks that needed to be done, but also of taking care of myself. I watched people in my support group also get better and better at the job—and so will you."

As an Alzheimer's caregiver, you've learned a lot—not only about Alzheimer's disease, but also about yourself. You now know that even though you may feel desperately alone, you are not alone. You now may realize that everyone—even those who say otherwise—took on the caregiver role with some reluctance. And that no one, even those who seem to be doing fine, can handle this illness without some difficulty. Caring for someone with Alzheimer's disease is a learning process from beginning to end.

# 26

# The Future: Is There Hope?

---- ❧ ----

Every year that goes by without an effective treatment for Alzheimer's disease, hundreds of thousands of new families must begin the difficult journey that you are facing or have been traveling. The National Institutes of Health projects that 360,000 new cases of Alzheimer's disease can be expected to develop each year and, as the baby-boomer generation ages, that number is expected to increase dramatically. If you are a child of someone with Alzheimer's, you may be especially fearful that you or your siblings will develop AD sometime later in life.

Is there hope for a treatment or a way to prevent Alzheimer's disease in the near future? Will a cure be developed in time to save you or others in your family from the fate of your parent? No one can say for certain, but there is more hope now than ever before. In the last few decades, there has been an explosion of research on the disease. This chapter will present an overview of some of the recent developments that might lead to an effective treatment or even a means of prevention in the next decade.

# Solving Dr. Alzheimer's Puzzle

The discovery of Alzheimer's disease occurred in 1906, when Dr. Alois Alzheimer did an autopsy on the brain of a deceased patient with severe dementia and found her brain riddled with two types of odd formations that he named tangles and plaques. At that time, Alzheimer assumed that either the tangles or the plaques or both together caused the dementia. What, however, causes the tangles and plaques to form? Today, scientists have learned a lot more about those tangles and plaques and are narrowing in on the puzzle of how they form in the brain and how to prevent or stop their formation.

## Tangles

Neurofibrillary tangles are the twisted and knotted remains of dead nerve cells found in the brains of people with Alzheimer's disease. The twisted or tangled parts of the nerve cell contain an abnormal form of a protein called tau. The more advanced the stage of the disease, the more tau deposits in the brain.

All protein molecules, like tau, carry out some essential process in cells, and if a protein is not normal, illness may result. The normal form of tau helps to support the axons of nerve cells—the parts of the cells that carry signals from one cell to another—and is critical to cell survival. When this protein becomes abnormal, as in the brains of those with Alzheimer's disease, it causes the tangles to form and the axons to shrivel up and die. Scientists don't yet know how or why the abnormal tau causes cells to die in those with AD.

## Plaques

The plaques that Dr. Alzheimer first discovered in the brain of his patient looked like bits of cellular debris. They had accumulated around dead nerve cells in the areas of the brain that affect memory and reasoning. In the 1980s, scientists discovered that the plaques were primarily composed of a molecular fragment of a larger protein found in healthy brains. The fragment is called beta-amyloid and the plaques are therefore referred to as beta-amyloid plaques, or simply amyloid plaques.

In 1984, a breakthrough was made in modern Alzheimer's disease research when scientists discovered that the amyloid protein that they isolated from the brain of a person with Down syndrome was the same as the protein in the plaques found in Alzheimer's disease. It was the first chemical evidence of a relationship between Down syndrome and Alzheimer's disease and it led to an explosion of new research. Scientists knew that Down syndrome was caused by a genetic abnormality before birth—people with the syndrome have an extra copy of chromosome 21. Could Alzheimer's disease also be linked to genetic factors and, if so, what genes are involved?

## Clues from Gene Research

The first place researchers began looking for genetic links to Alzheimer's was on chromosome 21, since that was the chromosome that affected Down syndrome. Sure enough, on chromosome 21, they found the gene for a larger protein of which the beta-amyloid protein found in plaques was a fragment. This larger protein was named amyloid-precursor protein or APP. In 1991, a mutant or defective form of the APP gene was discovered in the DNA of a family with hereditary early onset Alzheimer's—the first genetic link to AD to be discovered.

Not long thereafter, two more genes that give rise to early onset Alzheimer's disease were discovered—presenilin-1 and presenilin-2—located on chromosomes 14 and 1, respectively. Scientists have found more than 50 variations (alleles) of presenilin-1 and believe that variations in this gene account for about half the cases of early onset Alzheimer's disease. Variations in presenilin-2 have been found in just a few families with early onset Alzheimer's disease. Among persons without Down syndrome, variations in the APP gene on chromosome 21 lead to about 1 percent of the cases of early onset Alzheimer's disease.

Through testing the DNA of families with early onset AD, scientists had thus found three genes that were linked to the hereditary form of the disease. Unfortunately, these genes are dominant genes, meaning that a child who inherits any one of

Genes are like blueprints for proteins. Each gene has a code for how to make one protein or one part of a protein. Proteins are important because they are the chemicals that "get things done" in the body. For example, the melanin proteins give color to our hair and eyes. Hemoglobin proteins carry oxygen in our blood. Myosin proteins make our muscles move. Small differences between proteins can make them perform their action more efficiently or less efficiently. These differences between proteins, coded in the genes, cause the differences between individuals and even the differences between species of animals.

them from a parent will get Alzheimer's disease. As you know, however, less than 10 percent of the cases of AD are of the hereditary, or familial type. What about all of the cases of late onset, sporadic Alzheimer's?

In 1992, a researcher at Duke University discovered the first gene that affects late-onset AD—APOE$_4$ on chromosome 19. Everyone has some form of the APOE gene from each parent. APOE$_4$, one of the alleles or variations of this gene can cause an increased chance of developing AD when inherited from one parent and an even higher risk when inherited from both parents. Unlike the genes for early onset AD, this gene is a susceptibility gene, which means that not everyone with the gene will develop Alzheimer's. Several other genes, as well as environmental factors, may be involved in the development of late-onset AD.

In February 2001, two teams of scientists announced that they may soon isolate yet another susceptibility gene for late-onset Alzheimer's disease. The researchers believe this one lurks within a small region of chromosome 12.

Why all the rush to find genes that either cause or give a person with the gene a higher risk of developing Alzheimer's disease? Although proteins, hold the key to illness, genes hold the key to proteins, and the easiest way to discover the proteins involved in a disease is to discover the genes involved. Once the gene is known, the protein immediately becomes known as well and the design of a drug to somehow regulate it can begin. Once scientists know what protein is "sick," they can look for a medicine that either increases the amount of healthy protein or decreases or interferes with the unhealthy protein.

## Clues from Mice Models

Progress in effectively treating and preventing Alzheimer's disease had also been limited by the lack of an animal model for testing possible treatments. In recent years, however, new breakthroughs with mice have given scientists the kind of testing tool they need.

## Making a Mouse Sick

In 1996, scientists first genetically engineered mice to develop the memory loss characteristic of Alzheimer's disease. They inserted into mouse embryos the gene that increases production of the amyloid precursor protein or APP, which in turn caused plaques to develop in the brains of the mice similar to plaques found in the brains of humans with AD. The young mice then learned some memory-intensive tasks, such as navigating a maze. As the mice aged, they showed progressive memory loss similar to people with Alzheimer's disease.

Then, in 1999, other researchers were able to genetically engineer mice with the human gene coding for a form of the brain protein tau. In the study, scientists inserted human tau genes into mice. The mice later developed masses of abnormal tau filaments in nerve cells within their spinal cords, cortexes, and brain stems.

Finally, scientists have recently crossed the two types of genetically altered mice to create mice that have both plaques and tangles in their brains, thus modeling both abnormalities of the disease.

## A Promising Vaccine

Since the mid-1980s, many scientists have held the theory that it is the formation of the amyloid plaques that initiates the cell death that leads to the dementia symptoms of Alzheimer's disease. According to this theory, the tangles then form as a result of the accumulation of plaque formations.

Based on this theory, in 1999 researchers used the mice that had been genetically engineered to develop plaques and then immunized them with a drug called AN-1792. They hoped the drug would act as a vaccine and prevent the development of plaques in the brains of the mice. They were thrilled with the results. AN-1792 not only prevented new plaques from developing, it also significantly reduced existing plaques in the mice.

In late 2000, other scientists took the study of this vaccine another step. They showed that injecting the genetically altered mice with the vaccine not only removed the amyloid plaques in the brains of the mice, it also prevented the progressive memory loss and learning disabilities displayed by genetically altered mice that weren't vaccinated.

This is a tremendously exciting development for the treatment and prevention of Alzheimer's disease. Although mice and human beings have very different immune systems, if this vaccine works in humans the way it does in mice, it might actually stop the progression of Alzheimer's disease.

# Drugs

In addition to research on a vaccine for Alzheimer's, scientists are studying many new and old drugs and several herbal medicines as possible treatments. Currently, there are at least 19 new drugs in various phases of development. So far, as you saw in Chapter 5, "Dealing with the Bad News," the treatments that have been approved by the FDA are only helpful in about half of the cases of AD and only in the early to moderate stages of the disease.

The drugs currently in use are all in the category of acetylcholinesterase inhibitors, which are designed to increase the amount of acetylcholine, a substance that transmits nerve impulses across the synapses between nerve cells in the brain. People with Alzheimer's disease have lower levels of acetylcholine in their brains than healthy people. The idea behind this class of drugs is to increase the levels of acetylcholine in the brain in order to stimulate more nerve cell activity.

In addition to other drugs in this same class that might have more potency or fewer side effects, there also are drugs being developed and tested that work in different ways.

## Secretase Inhibitors—Memapsin 2

In the late 1990s, researchers discovered that two protein-cutting enzymes, (enzymes are proteins that act like catalysts), gamma secretase and beta secretase, play a role in the formation of amyloid plaques. These enzymes actually cut the fragment off the larger protein that becomes the beta-amyloid protein that forms the plaques. Beta secretase, which is also known as memapsin 2, is present in everyone's brains, not just

Alzheimer's patients. In healthy people, our bodies can dispose of the fragments these enzymes make at a normal rate. In Alzheimer's patients, however, they accumulate or pile up in the brain and form the plaques.

An inhibitor drug that would stop the action of these two enzymes would thus prevent the development of the plaques and stop the progression of Alzheimer's. In 2000, scientists created an inhibitor that effectively disabled memapsin 2. In test tube studies, this chemical inhibitor stops the production of beta-amyloid. If theorists are right and the amyloid plaques initiate Alzheimer's disease symptoms, then this substance, if developed into a safe and effective drug, would prevent and stop the progression of Alzheimer's. The memapsin 2 inhibitor still needs more testing in the laboratory, however, before it can be developed into a drug that can be tested on animals and humans.

## Anti-Inflammatories and OX2

Another characteristic of Alzheimer's disease, besides the development of plaques and tangles, is that the brains of those with the disease are chronically inflamed. The normal reaction to injury in the body is inflammation—swelling, redness, and heat—but in the central nervous system and the brain, that reaction is dulled in order to prevent damage to the brain. Scientists have recently discovered a protein, OX2, which is responsible for keeping the inflammatory processes in the brain more limited than in the rest of the body. In laboratory experiments, when OX2 was absent in mice and an injury was induced, the brain inflammation the mice suffered was greater and lasted longer.

This is very interesting for Alzheimer's research because it may well be the overactive inflammatory response in the brains of those with the disease that is responsible for the nerve damage and resulting dementia. If the inflammatory response either causes or contributes to the disease process, then nonsteroidal anti-inflammatory drugs such as ibuprofen may be able to protect against Alzheimer's disease. In 2001, a Phase II clinical trial will be testing the anti-inflammatory

———————— ❧ ————————

Work on the links between inflammation and Alzheimer's continues to be promising. A recent study compared the effects on a specific area of a rat's brain of short-term, high-dose injections of an inflammatory agent with the effects of longer-term, lower-doses of the agent. They found that both treatments were damaging, but that the chronic inflammation caused more damage to the nerve cells than did the short-term, intense inflammation. These results suggest that neuro-inflammation over a long period of time has the potential to cause some of the cellular damage seen in healthy aging, as well as in AD.

drug dapsone on Alzheimer's patients. Dapsone is a drug that has been used for decades in the treatment of leprosy.

Also in 2001 was the start of a large Phase II test of Rofecoxib, a COX-2 inhibitor, which is a new type of anti-inflammatory drug that produces fewer side effects than ibuprofen, and naproxen, a nonsteroidal anti-inflammatory that is the active ingredient in the over-the-counter drug Alleve. This is the first clinical trial to test two classes of anti-inflammatory drugs in patients with AD.

## Estrogen

Although it doesn't help those who already have Alzheimer's disease, estrogen may play a protective role in fighting dementia. In one study, researchers followed 1,124 post-menopausal women for five years and found that those who took estrogen had a 30 to 40 percent lower risk of developing Alzheimer's, and a later age of onset, than women who did not take the hormone. Scientists believe the benefits of estrogen are linked to its ability to increase cerebral blood flow. The hormone's effectiveness is currently being tested in much larger clinical studies. A significant problem with estrogen replacement therapy as a preventative treatment for Alzheimer's, however, is that synthetic estrogen increases a woman's chance of getting breast cancer by as much as 30 to 40 percent.

## Memantine

Currently, there are no FDA-approved drugs in the United States for the treatment of later-stage Alzheimer's disease. A drug that is available now only in Germany, memantine, may change that. A derivative of a decades-old anti-influenza drug, memantine has been used in Germany for over 10 years to treat Parkinson's disease and dementia, and to speed the recovery of comatose patients.

Memantine acts on the brain's N-methyl-D-aspartate (NMDA) receptors, which are among the structures that respond to glutamate, a specialized chemical messenger in the brain, like acetylcholine. The drug may block the chain reaction of events that lead to cell death.

A recent double-blind, placebo-controlled trial with more than 250 volunteers was conducted in the U.S. The study showed that memantine helped patients with moderately severe Alzheimer's to perform activities of daily living, such as dressing and bathing, more easily.

According to U.S. researchers, approval of memantine in Germany was based on studies that would not meet current U.S. Food and Drug Administration (FDA) standards. Because there is no drug specifically for Alzheimer's symptoms currently approved for individuals in the more severe stages of the disease, Alzheimer's advocates in the U.S. are hopeful that the FDA might approve memantine with as little as one additional favorable U.S. Phase III trial.

# Herbs

Although herbal medicine has not been studied as rigorously as conventional drugs for the treatment of Alzheimer's disease, some herbs that have been studied show promising results.

## Gingko, Ginseng, and Phosphatidyl Choline

Gingko is believed to increase the blood and oxygen flow to the brain, to improve metabolism, and to regulate the brain's neurotransmitters. People have long believed that gingko is good for mental functioning, but a recent study has shown that it is an effective treatment for Alzheimer's disease. The study was done to compare gingko special extract Egb761 with the four FDA-approved drugs currently used to treat Alzheimer's disease. Gingko was shown to be equally as effective as the cholinesterase inhibitor drugs in the treatment of mild to moderate Alzheimer's.

In addition to gingko, Panax ginseng, also known as Asian ginseng, has been shown to help improve memory. In one study, people who were given a combination of gingko and Panax ginseng showed increased ability to perform tests of cognitive performance.

Another herbal medicine that works in tandem with gingko is phosphatidyl choline, which is an important source of the neurotransmitter acetylcholine. Unlike with gingko alone, however, neither ginseng, phosphatidyl choline, nor combinations of these herbs have been clinically tested on Alzheimer's patients. With additional testing, these herbs may become useful in the treatment of the disease.

## Huperzine A

Another herbal medicine, huperzine A—which we mentioned in Chapter 5—is a drug-free acetylcholinesterase inhibitor, like the drugs currently approved to treat mild to moderate Alzheimer's disease. In both animal and clinical studies with humans, huperzine A has been shown to have a memory-boosting effect. Huperzine A has also been tested on Alzheimer's patients. In comparison studies with tacrine and Aricept (donepezil), two of the FDA-approved drugs for AD, huperzine A possessed a longer duration of action and the side effects were minimal.

## Sage

In England, researchers have studied the herb sage and found that it, like huperzine A, is an acetylcholinesterase inhibitor. Sage was often used in medieval herbals as a treatment that was "good for the brain." Although testing is only beginning in 2001 on Alzheimer's patients, the British researchers are quite hopeful that the herb will ultimately play some part in the treatment or prevention of Alzheimer's disease.

# Other Research Areas

Researchers have also been focusing on other types of brain research in the hopes of finding out more about Alzheimer's disease and other dementias.

## Brain Imaging Techniques

Since there is as yet no single, proven, laboratory diagnostic test for Alzheimer's disease, the current method of diagnosis combines physical and psychological testing with caregiver input and the doctor's judgment. Although this is reliable in over 90 percent of cases, a conclusive diagnosis is only possible with an autopsy done after the patient's death. Scientists are currently trying to develop and refine brain imaging techniques, such as magnetic resonance imaging (MRI) and computed tomography (CT) scanning to see if they can link early biological changes in the brain to changes in mental abilities and personality that are characteristic of Alzheimer's disease.

In 1999, researchers used a more powerful form of MRI called magnetic resonance microscopy (MRM) to detect amyloid plaques in brain tissue. They studied the autopsied brains of people both with and without Alzheimer's and were able to distinguish the plaques in the brains of those who had the disease. Scientists are hopeful that this technology may allow them to learn how the plaques develop in the brain, when an accumulation of the plaques begins to affect behavior, and whether or not they disappear with various treatments.

Not only might these sophisticated imaging techniques, as they continue to develop, provide doctors with a way to diagnose the disease earlier, they will also help scientists understand the pathology of the disease and develop new treatments.

## Reviving Brain Cells

Until recently, scientists thought that once nerve cells in the cerebral cortex of the brain—the center of higher intellectual functions—died, they could not be replaced and their function was gone forever. Now, however, researchers believe that the brain can produce new nerve cells for its learning and memory center, which could lead to new ways to treat people whose brains have been damaged by Alzheimer's and other diseases.

Several studies first demonstrated that in both mice and monkeys new cells can be regenerated in the hippocampus, the area of the brain associated with memory. In 1999, scientists traced the path followed by nerve cells in monkeys' brains that were created in one part of the brain and then migrated to the cerebral cortex. Once the new nerve cells arrive in the cerebral cortex, they become a new part of the brain's central circuitry. With mice, researchers found a way to restart the growth of brain cells by triggering a kind of "on-off" mechanism in the brain.

In 2000, researchers isolated stem cells—self-renewing cells that give rise to the more specialized cells of the human body—from human brains and demonstrated that these cells could develop into new brain cells. Then, in April 2001, doctors in San Diego, California, operated on a patient with Alzheimer's disease, injecting millions of her own genetically altered stem cells (from her skin) into her brain in the hopes that these cells would bring the atrophied cells in her brain back to life or stimulate the growth of new nerve cells. Assuming the procedure is not harmful, several other patients are expected to have similar operations later in 2001.

The possibility of stimulating new cell growth in the brain through surgery is extremely exciting. Although doctors will soon know whether or not the surgery has worked for the first patient, it may take years before they know if it will work for large numbers of Alzheimer's patients.

## Head Injuries

A new analysis of head injuries among World War II veterans has linked serious head injury in early adulthood with Alzheimer's disease in later life. The study also suggested that the more severe the head injury, the greater the risk of developing AD.

Although the new findings do not demonstrate a direct cause-and-effect relationship between head injury in early life and the development of Alzheimer's, they do show an association between the two that needs to be studied further. What scientists still need to learn is what is behind these findings—why head injury may be involved in AD and what may be happening biologically.

The increased risk of Alzheimer's disease as long as 50 years after a head injury has occurred is also an indication that AD is a chronic disease that unfolds over many decades. Understanding how a risk factor like head injury begins its destructive work early in life may ultimately lead to finding ways to interrupt the disease process at an earlier stage. Since an estimated 1.5 to 2 million individuals per year suffer a significant head injury in the United States, this could be an important environmental factor contributing to the development of AD.

## Glia Cells

The brain does not only have the hard-working nerve cells or neurons that send out the electrical signals that allow us to function, it also has another kind of cell—glia cells—that play an important role in brain functioning. Until recently, most research was focused on neurons, but scientists have now discovered that glia cells are equally essential to brain functioning. These cells forge and maintain the synapses—or contacts between nerve cells. It's possible that malfunctioning glia cells may play a role in brain disease such as Alzheimer's. The recent discovery of the role of glia cells has opened up yet another new path for research.

# Helping to Fund Hope

It has taken almost a century since Dr. Alzheimer's discovery of the disease for scientists to get close to finding an effective treatment for Alzheimer's disease. The recent strides in scientific research, particularly the genetic research that has been done in the last several decades, has helped scientists better understand many diseases, including Alzheimer's.

But, in addition to having new scientific tools, researchers have focused their attention on Alzheimer's disease rather than on other ailments because of the increased funding for and awareness of the disease in recent years that is a direct result of the work of nonprofit groups like the Alzheimer's Association.

The Alzheimer's Association is made up of family members of victims, who have been affected by this disease just as you have. Rather than allowing Alzheimer's to continue to devastate future generations, these caregivers and family members have decided to join together to fight for a cure. For you, too, now may be the time to give back to the Alzheimer's Association or another Alzheimer's organization for the support that you have gotten throughout your journey. In addition to the great benefit your help may provide other families who have been victimized by the disease, giving back to others can also be tremendously healing for you.

You can find opportunities to volunteer at the local office of an Alzheimer's group, or offer to lead a support group. Or, you can get involved in advocacy or fundraising for more research. You can do your part—however small—to bring even closer that day when a cure or vaccine is found. Perhaps even in your lifetime, Alzheimer's disease will become a thing of the past.

Although you've reached the end of this book, you may still have a long way to go on your journey as a caregiver. No matter where you are today on your journey, however, Alzheimer's disease has had an enormous effect on you. It has changed your life and, of course, the life of your loved one with AD. You will never be the same.

Dealing with the ravages of Alzheimer's disease has strengthened you in ways you never would have imagined. It has shown you the depths of empathy and compassion that you may not otherwise have known you had. You have learned about yourself and about life. All of this has happened not simply because of the disease, but because you faced the devastating diagnosis without turning your back or giving up. You are stronger, wiser, and more compassionate now—because you had the courage to care.

# Appendix A

## *Glossary*

**acetylcholine**   A neurotransmitter that seems to be involved in learning and memory and is deficient in the brains of people with Alzheimer's disease.

**activities of daily living (ADLs)**   Routine activities necessary for everyday life, such as eating, dressing, bathing, grooming, and toileting. People with Alzheimer's disease find it increasingly difficult to perform ADLs without assistance.

**Adult Day Care**   Programs that are generally available one to five days a week and provide participants with the opportunity to interact with others in a supportive environment, usually in a community center or facility.

**advance directives**   Written documents—which are completed and signed when a person is legally competent—that explain his or her medical wishes in advance, allowing an appointed representative to make treatment decisions for him or her at a later time.

**agnosia**   The inability to recognize or identify a familiar object or person. The person may think that a spoon is a key and try to open the door with it. This condition develops in the later stages of Alzheimer's and is the reason the affected person is not able to recognize people close to her.

**alleles**   Any variant form of a gene. For example, at the locus for eye color, a person might carry the allele for either blue or brown eyes.

**Alzheimer's disease** A progressive, degenerative disease of the brain characterized by the malfunctioning or death of nerve cells in several areas of the brain, which in turn causes the loss of mental abilities such as memory, comprehension, judgment, and reasoning.

**amino acid** The basic building blocks of proteins in the body. There are 20 amino acids necessary for human growth and function.

**anomia** The inability to find the right word for an object. This is characteristic of people in the early stages of Alzheimer's and may result in confusing or odd sentences.

**antibodies** Protein substances produced in the blood or tissues in response to a specific bacterium, virus, or other toxin. Antibodies destroy or weaken bacteria and neutralize organic poisons, and thus are the basis of the body's immune system.

**antioxidants** Nutrients present in fruits and vegetables and vitamin and mineral supplements that can prevent the damage caused by free radicals.

**aphasia** Partial or total loss of the ability to articulate ideas or comprehend spoken or written language, resulting from damage to the brain caused by injury or disease.

**apraxia** In the absence of motor or sensory impairment, total or partial loss of the ability to perform coordinated movements or manipulate objects.

**aromatherapy** A healing therapy that uses fragrant plant oils to benefit the body and mind. It has been shown to have a calming influence on Alzheimer's patients.

**beta amyloid protein** A type of protein found in humans which is abnormally processed by nerve cells in people with Alzheimer's disease and deposited in amyloid plaques in their brains.

**Binswanger disease** A type of dementia associated with stroke-related damage to the brain.

**biological marker or biomarker** The measure of a biological process, such as levels of a protein in blood or spinal fluid, to aid in the diagnosis and treatment of a disease.

**body language** Aspects of nonverbal communication, including facial expressions and gestures, which convey underlying emotions or feelings. People with Alzheimer's disease are very sensitive to body language and all nonverbal communication.

**cardiopulmonary resuscitation (CPR)** An emergency procedure, often employed after cardiac arrest, in which cardiac massage, artificial respiration, and drugs are used to maintain the circulation of oxygenated blood to the brain.

**catastrophic reactions** An extreme emotional overreaction to a situation. For persons with AD, catastrophic reactions can include changes in mood, stubbornness, hostile or violent reactions, cursing, and abusive behavior.

**cholinesterase inhibitors** Drugs that delay or inhibit the breakdown of acetylcholine in the brain.

**chromosome** A threadlike, linear strand of DNA and associated proteins in the nucleus of animal and plant cells that carries the genes and functions in the transmission of hereditary information.

**clinical trials** Organized, controlled studies that test whether a drug or other treatment is safe and effective in humans.

**companionship services** Services that provide people who visit the home and offer companionship as well as supervision and personal care to ill or homebound people.

**conservatorship (or guardianship)** A legal designation by a court which, after evidence of a patient's incompetence, allows a conservator to control and manage a patient's finances.

**cortex** A thin coating of nerve cells covering the surfaces of the brain's two hemispheres. It controls many behaviors including interpreting sensory information, intellectual abilities, and emotional reactions.

**Creutzfeldt-Jakob disease** A rare infectious disease that causes memory failure and behavioral changes.

**CT (computed tomography) scan**  An imaging technique that shows the internal structure of the brain and helps to diagnose brain tumors and small strokes.

**custodial care**  Care that focuses on supervision and assistance rather than on efforts to heal or cure.

**delusion**  A false belief, idea, or story that is firmly maintained despite all evidence to the contrary. People with AD often have delusions that people are out to harm them in some way even though there are no facts to support these beliefs.

**dementia**  Symptoms of mental deterioration severe enough to interfere with a person's daily functioning, including loss of intellectual abilities, as well as changes in personality, mood, and behavior. Alzheimer's disease is the most common cause of dementia.

**Down syndrome**  A syndrome that causes slowed growth, abnormal facial features, and mental retardation. Most people with Down syndrome develop Alzheimer's disease in adulthood.

**durable power of attorney (DPA)**  A legal document that allows an individual to authorize an agent to make legal decisions when he or she is no longer able to do so. There are DPAs for property and for healthcare. The latter allows a person to appoint an agent to make decisions regarding healthcare.

**early onset Alzheimer's disease**  When symptoms of Alzheimer's disease appear before age 60 or 65. This occurs in less than 10 percent of patients and is usually associated with a genetic or hereditary pre-disposition to the disease.

**Electroencephalogram (EEG)**  A test that measures the brain's electrical activity.

**endorphins**  A group of hormones found mainly in the brain that bind to certain receptors, ultimately reducing the sensation of pain and positively affecting the emotions.

**enzyme**  A specialized protein that acts as a catalyst, speeding up chemical reactions within a cell.

**familial Alzheimer's disease**   The rarer form of Alzheimer's that runs in families.

**fecal impaction**   A condition that occurs when the feces are too hard and they block the rectum.

**free radicals**   Highly toxic molecules in your body capable of causing damage in brain and other tissue. A meat-based, high-fat diet can increase the number of free radicals in the body. Smoking also floods the body with free radicals.

**gene**   A hereditary unit that occupies a specific location on a chromosome and carries a code for making a protein, which then creates a particular characteristic in an organism. Genes have many different forms and can undergo mutations, which can lead to illness.

**guided imagery or visualization**   The process of forming a set of mental pictures or images to aid in healing, alleviate physical conditions, or achieve goals.

**hallucination**   Hearing, seeing, feeling, tasting, or smelling something that does not really exist, except in the mind of the person experiencing it. Hallucinations are often the result of a misperception of something in the environment.

**hippocampus**   An area of the brain that has a central role in memory.

**home health aides**   People who provide personal care to patients at home and assist with light household tasks.

**homemaker or housekeeping services**   Services that provide various household assistance, including shopping, laundry, cleaning, and meal preparation.

**hospice care**   A program that treats the emotional, spiritual, social, and financial needs of terminally ill patients in an inpatient facility or in the patient's home.

**immune system**   The system of the body containing organs, cell tissue, and cell products, such as antibodies, that differentiates the self from foreign substances and then neutralizes the potentially harmful foreign organisms or substances, protecting the body from disease.

**inflammation** A complex protective response of the body that causes redness, warmth, swelling, and tenderness. Inflammation often goes along with vigorous action of the immune system.

**late-onset Alzheimer's disease** The most common form of Alzheimer's disease. It usually strikes after age 65 and may or may not be hereditary.

**Lewy body dementia** A dementing illness with symptoms similar to Parkinson's and characterized by protein deposits called Lewy bodies.

**lumbar puncture** (also called a spinal tap) A test in which a needle is used to withdraw cerebrospinal fluid that surrounds the spinal cord. It is used in the diagnosis of infections, tumors, and other conditions.

**Medic Alert Program** A program that distributes identification bracelets, which in turn provide medical information in case of an emergency.

**meditation** A technique for quieting the mind and relaxing the body, with the goals of getting in touch with feelings or reaching deeper levels of contemplation.

**metabolic diseases** Diseases that alter or interfere with the normal concentration of various substances in the blood. Several metabolic diseases can cause dementia.

**mirror** A term used to describe behavior which mimics or copies the behavior of the person with whom a person is interacting. People with Alzheimer's disease often mimic the tone or emotional state of the person who is talking with them.

**MRI (magnetic resonance imaging)** A scanning technique that can reveal small molecular changes in the brain, as well as the contrast between normal and abnormal tissue.

**multi-infarct disease (MID) or vascular dementia** A disease in which repeated strokes damage brain cells, ultimately causing dementia. The disease is sometimes treatable and usually has an abrupt onset.

**neurofibrillary tangles** Twisted nerve cell fibers found in the brains of Alzheimer's patients.

**neurotransmitter** A chemical substance that conducts electrical impulses from one nerve cell to another. There are several kinds of neurotransmitters in the body, most of which we know very little about.

**normal pressure hydrocephalus** A buildup of cerebrospinal fluid on the brain that causes symptoms of dementia.

**ombudsperson** A person who investigates and mediates settlements, especially between consumers and an institution or company. There are ombudspersons specializing in helping people find and evaluate nursing facilities.

**ophthalmologist** A medical doctor who deals with the anatomy, functions, pathology, and treatment of the eye and eye diseases.

**palliative care** Care that focuses on ways to relieve or soothe symptoms and make life better for people who are dying without attempting to cure them. With palliative care, death and dying are viewed as a natural occurrence.

**parietal lobe** The area of the brain that lies beneath each parietal bone and controls functions such as language comprehension and aspects of time and space orientation.

**Parkinson's disease** A degenerative disease characterized by damage to nerve cells in certain parts of the brain. Symptoms include muscle stiffness, tremors, speech impediments, and sometimes dementia.

**Pick's disease** A relatively rare form of dementia that affects the part of the brain known as the frontal lobe. It causes dramatic changes in personality, but does not initially affect memory.

**plaques (neuritic plaques or amyloid plaques)** Clusters of abnormal deposits of "amyloid"—a kind of protein—mixed with fragments of dead or dying nerve cells found in the brains of Alzheimer's patients.

**pressure sores (decubitus ulcers)**   Sores that develop on parts of the body when a person is confined without movement to a bed or to a chair for long periods of time.

**protein**   A family of large natural chemicals in the body that are fundamental components of all cells. All protein molecules carry out some essential process for the growth and repair of tissue, and if a protein is not normal, illness may result.

**relaxation exercise**   A mental exercise that relaxes the body and helps to relieve tension and stress.

**respite care**   Services that provide relief to caregivers by offering short-term, temporary care in the home or in a facility.

**rummaging**   A behavior, common in people with AD, that involves going through closets, drawers, or other containers as though searching for something.

**Safe Return Program**   The Alzheimer's Association's nationwide identification, support, and registration program that assists in the safe return of people with AD who are lost.

**serotonin**   A neurotransmitter in the brain. The concentration of serotonin is usually reduced in the brains of Alzheimer's patients.

**skilled nursing care**   A level of care that includes ongoing medical and nursing services in the treatment of injury or disease provided by licensed nurses.

**SPECT (single photon emission computed tomography) scan**   A brain imaging technique that measures blood flow through various parts of the brain in order to identify changes in the brain.

**sporadic Alzheimer's disease**   Nonhereditary Alzheimer's disease, the most common form of the disease.

**stages**   The course of a disease's progression or level as defined by how severe the symptoms are at any point. Alzheimer's disease is often described in three stages: early, moderate, and late or severe.

**stem cells** Self-renewing cells that give rise to the more specialized cells of the human body, such as muscle cells, blood cells, and brain cells.

**stroke** Brain damage from either the rupturing of a blood vessel in the brain (cerebral hemorrhage) or the blockage of blood vessels in the brain (cerebral infarction).

**subdural hematoma** A collection of blood resulting from trauma to a blood vessel located below the "dura mater," a membrane that lines the outside of the brain and spinal cord. Subdural hematomas are surgically treatable.

**sundowning** Confused behavior which occurs in the late afternoon or early evening.

**tau protein** The major protein that makes up neurofibrillary tangles found in degenerating nerve cells.

**temporal lobe** The area of the brain that contains the sensory center of hearing, as well as other sensory, interpretative, and problem-solving functions.

**TIAs (transient ischemic attacks)** Mini-strokes which occur when an internal blood clot temporarily blocks an already narrowed artery in the brain and then dissolves on its own.

**vaccine** A preparation of a modified or weakened bacterium or virus that is used to stimulate the body's antibody production against the virus or bacterium, but is incapable of causing severe infection itself.

**visualization** See guided imagery.

**wandering** A common behavior of people with Alzheimer's disease, who walk or wander away from familiar locations and get lost.

# Appendix B

## *Further Reading*

There are many books on Alzheimer's disease. Some are focused more on caring for someone with Alzheimer's, and are written for either the family caregiver or the professional caregiver or both. Others tell personal stories of people with Alzheimer's, and still others are more medically oriented and attempt to describe the pathology of the disease and recent research. There are also books by people who have Alzheimer's disease.

Each of the books has something to offer, depending on the information you are looking for. The following list is not comprehensive. Most of the general books cover the kind of information you have read in this book—with more or less detail on certain issues. I've tried to include some of the general books I think are best, as well as books in other categories, such as memoirs or personal accounts. Many of these are wonderful moving stories by caregivers and patients.

The Alzheimer's Association also publishes very useful literature, including articles, newsletters, flyers, and pamphlets on various aspects of the disease or caregiving. To get a list of the publications of the Alzheimer's Association, call their national office at 1-800-272-3900 and ask for the publications catalog. See Appendix C, "Community Resources," for a list of other organizations and community resources that might also publish useful literature.

# General Books

Andresen, Gayle. *Caring for People with Alzheimer's Disease.* Baltimore: Health Professions Press, 1995.

Aronson, M. K., ed. *Understanding Alzheimer's Disease: What It Is, How to Cope with It, Future Directions.* New York: Hungry Minds, 1988.

Castleman, Michael, Dolores Gallagher-Thompson, Ph.D., and Matthew Naythons, M.D. *There's Still a Person in There: The Complete Guide to Treating and Coping with Alzheimer's.* New York: Putnam, 1999.

Cohen, D., and C. Eisdorfer. *The Loss of Self: A Family Resource for the Care of Alzheimer's Disease and Related Disorders.* New York: Norton, 1986.

Cohen, Elwood. *Alzheimer's Disease: Prevention, Intervention, and Treatment.* Lincolnwood, IL: NTC/Contemporary Publishing Group, 1999.

Coughlin, Patricia. *Facing Alzheimer's.* New York: Ballantine Books. 1993.

Gray-Davidson, Frena. *The Alzheimer's SourceBook for Caregivers: A Practical Guide for Getting Through the Day.* Los Angeles: Lowell House, 1996.

Gruetzner, Howard. *Alzheimer's: A Caregiver's Guide and SourceBook.* New York: John Wiley & Sons, Inc., 1992.

Hay, Jennifer. *Alzheimer's and Dementia: Questions You Have ... Answers You Need.* Allentown, PA: People's Medical Society, 1996.

Jones, Moyra. *Gentle Care: Changing the Experience of Alzheimer's Disease in a Positive Way.* Point Roberts, WA: Hartley and Marks, 1999.

Kuhn, Daniel. *Alzheimer's Early Stages: First Steps in Caring and Treatment.* Alameda, CA: Hunter House, 1999.

Mace, Nancy L., and Peter Rabins. *The 36-Hour Day: A Family Guide to Caring for Persons with Alzheimer Disease, Related Dementing Illnesses, and Memory Loss in Later Life.* Baltimore: Johns Hopkins University Press, 1991.

Markin, R. *The Alzheimer's Cope Book: The Complete Care Manual for Patients and Their Families.* Secaucus, NJ: Citadel Press, 1992.

Medina, John. *What You Need to Know About Alzheimer's.* Oakland, CA: CME, Inc., and New Harbinger, 1999.

Nelson, James Lindemann, and Hilde Lindemann Nelson. *Alzheimer's: Answers to Hard Questions for Families.* New York: Doubleday, 1996.

Powell, Lenore S., and Katie Courtice. *Alzheimer's Disease: A Guide for Families.* New York: Addison Wesley, 1992.

Raymond, Florian. *Surviving Alzheimer's: A Guide for Families.* Forest Knolls, CA: Elder Books, 1996.

Rob, Caroline. *The Caregiver's Guide.* Boston: Houghton Mifflin, 1991.

Sheridan, Carmel. *Failure-Free Activities for the Alzheimer's Patient.* Forest Knolls, CA: Elder Books, 1987.

Warner, Mark L. *The Complete Guide to Alzheimer's Proofing Your Home.* West Lafayette, IN: Purdue University Press, 1998.

## Personal Stories

Bayley, John. *Elegy for Iris.* New York: St. Martin's Press, 1999.

Doernberg, M. *Stolen Mind: The Slow Disappearance of Ray Doernberg.* Chapel Hill, NC: Algonquin Books, 1989.

Grubbs, William M. *In Sickness & in Health: Caring for a Loved One with Alzheimer's.* Forest Knolls, CA: Elder Books, 1997.

Honel, R. W. *Journey with Grandpa: Our Family's Struggle with Alzheimer's Disease*. Baltimore: John Hopkins University Press, 1988.

McGowin, Diana Friel. *Living in the Labyrinth: A Personal Journey Through the Maze of Alzheimer's*. New York: Delacorte Press, 1993.

Shanks, Lela Knox. *A Caregiver's Guide to Alzheimer's*. Lincoln, NE: University of Nebraska Press, 1996.

Zabbia, K. H. *Painted Diaries: A Mother and Daughter's Experience Through Alzheimer's*. Minneapolis: Fairview Press, 1996.

# Appendix C

## *Community Resources*

## Organizations and Community Resources on Alzheimer's Disease

### The Alzheimer's Association

The largest national voluntary health organization committed to finding a cure for Alzheimer's and helping those affected by the disease. The Alzheimer's Association has chapters in every state. To find the nearest chapter to you call the toll-free number or visit its Web site at www.alz.org for a list of local chapters. The national office is located at:

919 North Michigan Avenue, Suite 1100
Chicago, Illinois 60611-1676
Phone: 312-335-8700 or 1-800-272-3900
Fax: 312-335-1110

### Alzheimer's Disease Education and Referral Center (ADEAR)

The ADEAR Center is a service of the federal government's National Institute on Aging (NIA). It was established in 1990 and provides information about Alzheimer's disease, its impact on families and health professionals, and research into possible causes and cures. By calling the toll-free number, you may speak with an information specialist who will answer questions about Alzheimer's disease or provide information about the latest research findings on Alzheimer's disease, including studies on new treatments. You can also order publications about Alzheimer's disease and locate other groups to contact for more information, publications, and services.

PO Box 8250
Silver Springs, MD 20907
1-800-438-4380

## Alzheimer's Disease Centers in the United States

Also funded through the National Institute on Aging, these centers conduct research, offer educational programs for professional and family caregivers, and operate memory disorder clinics. They can refer you to other clinics and services if you do not live near any of them. Also, the National Institute on Aging funds a consortium of more than 30 centers nationwide devoted to clinical drug trials known as the Alzheimer's Disease Cooperative Study. You can contact them at:

8950 Villa La Jolla Drive, Suite 2200
La Jolla, CA 92037
619-622-5880
www.alz.ucsd.edu

Several states, such as Florida, California, and Illinois, fund memory disorder clinics, so check with the state Department of Public Health to see if your state has such facilities. Your local chapter of the Alzheimer's Association will also be able to direct you to other Alzheimer's disease centers at academic medical centers and other specialists in your area.

## Other Helpful Organizations

Many other organizations that are not specifically devoted to Alzheimer's disease can provide you with useful information and services at various stages in the person with Alzheimer's disease. The titles of most of the following organizations are usually self-explanatory. They include:

**The American Association of Homes and Services for the Aging**
901 E Street, N.W., Suite 500
Washington, DC 20004-2037
202-783-2242

An organization that provides information about and lobbies for nonprofit nursing homes.

**The American Health Care Association**
1201 L Street, N.W.
Washington, DC 20005
202-842-4444

An organization whose members include both for-profit and nonprofit nursing homes.

**American Association for Geriatric Psychiatry**
7910 Woodmont Avenue, Suite 1350
Bethesda, MD 20814-3004
301-654-7850

**American Geriatrics Society**
770 Lexington Avenue, Suite 400
New York, NY 10021
212-308-1414

**American Association of Retired Persons**
601 E Street, NW
Washington, DC 20049
202-434-2277 or 1-800-424-3410

**Children of Aging Parents**
1609 Woodbourne Road, Suite 302A
Levittown, PA 19057
215-945-6900 or 1-800-227-7294

**Department of Veteran Affairs**
810 Vermont Avenue, NW
Washington, DC 20420
202-628-3030 or 1-800-827-1000

**Eldercare Locator**
1-800-677-1116

**Family Survival Project**
425 Bush Street, #500
San Francisco, CA 94108
415-434-3388 or 1-800-445-8106

**Help for Incontinent People**
PO Box 544
Union, SC 29379
1-800-252-3337

**Hospice Helpline**
National Hospice Organization
1901 N Moore Street, Suite 901
Arlington, VA 22209
1-800-658-8898

**Legal Counsel for the Elderly**
American Association of Retired Persons
601 E Street, NW
Washington, DC 20049
1-800-424-3410

**Long Term Care Ombudsman Program**
PO Box 126 (21 Bangor Street)
Augusta, ME 04332-0216
207-621-1079 (Augusta area) or 1-800-499-0229
Fax: 207-621-0509

**Medicare Hotline**
1-800-638-6833
In Maryland: 1-800-492-6603

**National Association for Hispanic Elderly**
3325 Wilshire Boulevard
Los Angeles, CA 90010
213-487-1922

**National Association for Home Care**
519 C Street NE, Stanton Park
Washington, DC 20002
202-547-7424

**National Association of Area Agencies on Aging**
(Native American)
1112 16th Street NW, Suite 100
Washington, DC 20036

**National Association of Interfaith Volunteer Caregivers**
368 Broadway, Suite 103
Kingston, NY 12401
914-331-1358 or 1-800-350-7438

**National Association of Social Workers**
750 First Street NE
Washington, DC 20002
202-408-8600

**National Caucus and Center on Black Aged**
1424 K Street NW, Suite 500
Washington, DC 20005
202-637-8400

**National Citizens Coalition for Nursing Home Reform**
1424 16th Street NW, Suite 202
Washington, DC 20036-2211
202-332-2275
www.nccnhr.org

**The National Counsel on Aging**
NIAD 409 Third Street
Washington, DC 20024
202-479-1200

**National Family Caregivers Association**
10400 Connecticut Avenue, #500
Kensington, MD 20895-3944
1-800-896-3650
www.nfcacares.org
E-mail: info@nfcacares.org

**National Funeral Directors Association**
11121 West Oklahoma Avenue
Milwaukee, WI 53227
414-541-2500 or 1-800-228-6332

**Older Women's League**
666 11th Street, NW, Suite 700
Washington, DC 20001
1-800-825-3695

In addition to the federal National Institute on Aging, each state has some sort of agency devoted to helping senior citizens. Some of those agencies may have useful information or services for you as an Alzheimer's caregiver.

# Appendix D

## *Online Resources*

The Internet is a great place to learn about Alzheimer's disease, keep up on the latest research, and get support for your role as a caregiver. Because the Internet changes so fast, some of the following Web sites may no longer be operating or the addresses may have changed. When the Web site is for an organization already listed in Appendix C, "Community Resources," I have just listed the Web address here. When the Web site is for an organization that is only reachable online, I've described the site.

**Alzheimer's Association**
www.alz.org

**Alzheimer's Disease Education and Referral Center**
www.alzheimers.org

**Alzheimers.com**
www.alzheimers.com

The editorial staff of Alzheimers.com, led by Michael Castleman, author of a book on Alzheimer's, screens the latest news and research on Alzheimer's, reviews the hundreds of Alzheimer's-related sites on the Internet, and provides an interactive forum for people with Alzheimer's disease. The site is published by PlanetRx.

**AlzheimerSupport.com**
www.alzheimersupport.com

This site serves Alzheimer's disease sufferers by reporting the latest news in Alzheimer's disease treatment and research. It also sells nutritional supplements and donates profits from each purchase to Alzheimer's disease research.

### Alzheimer's Disease-All You Need to Know
www.agelessdesign.com

A site by Mark L. Warner, the author of *The Complete Guide to Alzheimer's Proofing Your Home*. The site provides a free Alzheimer's newsletter, links, and resources, and sells the book.

### Alzheimer's Disease at Suite101.com
www.suite101.com/welcome.cfm/alzheimers_disease

This site publishes bi-weekly articles about Alzheimer's disease, updated links, news, informal polls, moderated discussion, Alzheimer's support board.

### Alzheimer's Outreach
alzheimers.zarcrom.com

This site offers numerous directories on various aspects of Alzheimer's disease.

### Alzheimer's Chat Room
www.alzheimerschat.com

This site provides an Alzheimer's disease chat room, as well as message boards.

### Alzheimer's Disease International
www.alz.co.uk/

The site for an umbrella organization of national Alzheimer's Associations around the world.

### Alzheimer's Disease—Caregivers Speak Out
www.chpublishers.com/

A site focusing on helping caregivers better understand Alzheimer's disease and learn compassionate communication with those who have the disease.

**Alzheimer's Disease Medical Information**

www.mediconsult.com/alzheimers/

A virtual medical clinic offering medical and drug information and support groups on Alzheimer's disease and other long-term medical conditions.

**Alzheimer's Disease**

alzheimers.about.com

A site with directories for various topics related to this disease, including caregiving, research, nursing home issues, and behavioral problems. Also includes a drug index, weekly newsletter, support, and forum.

**Alzheimer's Disease Community**

community.healingwell.com/community/scripts/
community.pl?ClientID

This site provides message boards and chat for caregivers dedicated to sharing information, support, and coping strategies to deal with Alzheimer's disease.

**Alzheimer's Disease Research**

www.ahaf.org/alzdis/about/adabout.htm

The site for a program to fund research and educate the public about Alzheimer's disease.

**Alzheimer's Disease Resource Center at HealingWell.com**

www.healingwell.com/alzheimers/

Medical news, information, chat, articles, books, message boards, and a directory of related sites on Alzheimer's disease.

**Alzheimer's Resource Center**

www.mayohealth.org/mayo/common/htm/alzheimers.htm

The Mayo Clinic site offers information, explanations, and advice about treatment and care for patients with Alzheimer's disease.

### Alzheimer's Disease Videos
www.alzheimersvideo.com/

A site that sells videos for Alzheimer's disease caregivers and patients, including calming, relaxing nature videos.

### Alzheimer Store
thealzheimerstore.com

Products for families and caregivers for the treatment of Alzheimer's disease.

### The ALZwell Home Page
www.alzwell.com/

This large, comprehensive site contains address and telephone resources and information on legal issues. It also includes donation information, stories, and tips for caregivers.

### Alois Alzheimer Center
www.alois.com

A site dedicated to the care, treatment, and study of Alzheimer's disease.

### American Health Assistance Foundation
www.ahaf.org

Funds research on Alzheimer's disease and provides financial assistance to patients and caregivers.

### Caregiver Support
www.nymemory.org/devig/carsup.html

Information on techniques for caregivers of patients with Alzheimer's disease. FAQs from caregivers. Assessment and treatment of caregivers.

### Caregiver Survivor Resources
www.caregiver911.com

This site focuses on general caregiver support and assistance.

## Mr. Long-Term Care
www.mrltc.com/

Provides long-term-care news and information. Includes resources for Parkinson's, Alzheimer's, heart disease, and other long-term illnesses.

## The National Citizens' Coalition for Nursing Home Reform
www.nccnhr.org

## The National Family Caregivers Association
www.nfcacares.org/

## Painted Diaries: Two Women and Alzheimer's
www.alzheimersart.net

Painted Diaries is a place for Alzheimer's caregivers to submit stories from their caregiving experiences, as well as read about two women's struggles with the disease.

## U.S. Resources: Alzheimer's Disease etc.—Internet Aging Resources
www.aoa.dhhs.gov/jpost/us-ad.html

The site maintained by the U.S. Administration on Aging provides a guide to resources on AD and dementia.

## Well Spouse Foundation
www.wellspouse.org

A site for well spouses who face the problems of anger, guilt, fear, isolation, grief, and financial need.

## A Year to Remember ... with My Mother and Alzheimer's Disease
www.zarcrom.com/users/yeartorem/

A comprehensive site developed by a woman whose mother had Alzheimer's disease. It has articles for caregivers as well as poems, photos, a caregiver's journal, and stories. It also provides a message board, links, and resources.

# Index

# About the Author

───────────────── ❧ ─────────────────

A successful author and screenwriter, **Joanne Parrent** majored in American Culture at the University of Michigan and received her degree in Communications from UCLA. She began her career in the film industry, writing, producing, and directing documentary films. Among her credits in the documentary field is *The Healing Force*, a feature-length documentary released in theaters, about Norman Cousins' remarkable recovery from a life-threatening illness. Parrent has written dramatic screenplays for Walt Disney Productions and Bette Midler's All Girl Productions, mini-series for PBS, and series television, including the CBS hit *Dr. Quinn, Medicine Woman*.

Parrent is the author of four nonfiction books and has edited several other published books. Among her books are *Life After Johnnie Cochran* (HarperCollins, 1995), *Once More with Feeling* (Dove Books, 1997), and *You'll Never Make Love in This Town Again* (Dove Books, 1996). The latter was on *The New York Times* and *Los Angeles Times* bestseller lists for over four months. In the late 1970s, Parrent was an editor of *Chrysalis*, a women's art and literary magazine. At that time she also served on the board of The Woman's Building, a space for women artists and writers.